"Fun, witty and chockfull of useful suggestions, thi Abigail Wurf provides an insider's perspective on shares tried and true ways for getting through the read for anyone with ADHD!"

Laurie Dupar
PMHNP, RN, PCC

"Forget Perfect is a reader-friendly book that addresses the core issues facing adults with ADHD. Jam-packed with concrete examples, common sense recommendations and coaching tips, it will help the reader move forward step-by-step toward success."

Jodi Sleeper-Triplett, MCC, SCAC, BCC
JST Coaching & Training

"The subtitle says it all: How to Succeed in Your Profession and Personal Life Even if You Have ADHD. *Abigail Wurf has condensed years of personal and professional experience into a book that covers much of what a person with ADD or ADHD needs to know to successfully navigate a world where often the seemingly little things can often present the biggest problems. This is an easy-to-read, how-to-coach-yourself-to-success handbook for adults with ADD/ADHD. It is also a good read for anyone who lives or works with an adult with ADD/ADHD. This book will help a lot of people, and I am recommending it to everyone!"*

Sarah D. Wright
Author of *Fidget to Focus and ADHD Coaching Matters: The Definitive Guide.*

"Readers will experience immediate, welcome relief with the title alone! Forget Perfect clearly suggests that the misconception many hold that "EVERYONE ELSE IS PERFECT" can be dispelled forever! Abigail Wurf has contributed a fresh "How to..." for living more effectively with ADHD, and includes steps to achieve this goal. It's one thing to state that we all need to "communicate more clearly at work," and quite another to outline concrete options that drive home the point. Bravo to Ms. Wurf on this achievement!"

Wilma Fellman, M.Ed., LPC
Career & Life Planning Counselor, Author, ADHD Coach Trainer

Forget Perfect

How to Succeed in Your Profession and Personal Life Even If You Have ADHD!

Abigail Wurf, M.Ed, PCC

Slow Bell Press

Dedication

For my mother, Mildred Kiefer Wurf. You've listened to me, supported me, and cheered me on. The sheer number of hours you have helped on this and other projects cannot be counted, nor can the unabated belief you have continued to have in me. It humbles me. It might sound like a cliché, but I won the mom lottery!

Slow Bell Press
The Towers
Washington, D.C
www.abigailwurf.com

ISBN: 978-0996140607

First Edition

Printed in the United States of America

Table of Contents

Preface

My own journey with ADHD started at an early age. I was easily distracted, hyperactive (I talked compulsively), had difficulty with memorization and learning to read. Then as a teenager I struggled with depression. The diagnosis came later.

I was 30 years old. I had been a professional dancer and choreographer, as well as a dance teacher and co-owner of a dance studio. After numerous painful injuries, seeing many doctors, and undergoing several surgeries and grueling periods of rehabilitation, it was clear that pain would follow me the rest of my life. I needed to move in another direction and decided to go to graduate school.

I had struggled with learning disabilities while in school so I was re-tested for these as part of my graduate school application process. Over the course of the testing, I was diagnosed with ADHD.

This diagnosis changed my life. It explained my failures and struggles and set me on a new path. Medication, as well as therapy and coaching, helped me turn my life around. I learned that it was possible to be on time and get things done. In the process of learning to manage my ADHD, I found my second career as an ADHD coach, a career that is profoundly satisfying to me. What I learned and continue to learn from dealing with ongoing physical pain and with my ADHD symptoms is that I can manage just about anything. I am strong. Maybe not physically, but mentally. And I am strong because of my experiences.

It is what I've learned from these experiences and my ADHD coaching that I share with you. If you have struggled too, and I know many of you have, the fact that you are picking up this book means that you believe your life can change. At some level you have hope that you can live in an easier manner, and more aligned with your values, interests, and strengths. I believe you can too.

Is ADHD a Gift?

If you have been diagnosed with ADHD or suspect you have it, is this a "gift" or a disability? The ADHD community differs over whether to consider ADHD a gift. One faction believes ADHD should be presented as a gift because doing so builds self-esteem. The other faction considers ADHD a disability.

Your life's journey will be discovering what you can do and learning how to work around the obstacles having ADHD presents.

The gift group, in focusing on the tendency of individuals with ADHD to be creative, is trying to build the self-esteem of people diagnosed with ADHD, especially those young people who have had their esteem battered by negative experiences in life resulting from their undiagnosed ADHD. While this stance is put forward with good intentions, it sets up false expectations. These young people are going to find out that the world has plenty of creative people who don't have ADHD. They will find out that this gift means working harder and longer battling attention deficit and lack of motivation.

I consider ADHD a disability and I propose acknowledging it as a disability, not an excuse. Like anyone, you do the best you can with what you have. Your life's journey will be discovering what you can do and how to work around the obstacles having ADHD presents. My hope is through your journey you will figure out what you want to do and then to go full steam ahead after that dream.

Diagnosis and Treatment for ADHD

You can move forward only when you get the professional help and support you need. An important initial step is getting a diagnosis. While ADHD cannot be cured, there are effective treatments for ADHD that help you manage your symptoms. A multi-modal treatment or multi-pronged approach is the most effective.

Getting Diagnosed

If you think you have ADHD, get a diagnosis to see if you are a candidate for medication. Get an appointment with a psychiatrist to get that diagnosis. The reason for this is that psychiatrists (unlike psychologists) can prescribe medication, which works for 70% of the people who try them. You may have to work with your psychiatrist and try one or more different medications until you find the right one for you. It took me trying three or four until we found the best combination of medication and dosage.

Multimodal Treatment Plan

I think of the multi-modal treatment plan for people affected by ADHD as the "Hand Plan." It includes five things, listed in no particular order:

- *Psychiatrist (for prescriptions and therapy, if they do it)*
- *Coach, therapist, and/or social worker*
- *Medication (if it works for you)*
- *Exercise plan (check with your doctor first)*
- *Good sleep*

In this book I discuss coaching, exercise, and sleep and advocate for considering medication to support coaching or therapy for ADHD. Appendix A provides more detailed information on multimodal treatment for ADHD.

While many think of treatment as something done to or for you, managing your ADHD symptoms calls on you to take actions that change how you live your life and shift attitudes you likely have been carrying with you most of your life. Don't delay. The time to start is now.

Forget Perfect!

One of the reasons those of us with ADHD don't start on something, especially pursuing the life we want, is because we know that whatever we start will not be perfect in the end. Or we are constantly judging ourselves against the ideal of perfection and feeling we come up short. As a result, we believe we can't win, can't succeed at anything. And often we don't even bother trying. My gift to you is this: let go of the notion of perfection. All it brings is self-doubt, frustration, and grief.

The best way to go after the life you want is to Forget Perfect! Simply let go of the idea of perfection. Stop wasting your precious time trying to make everything just right. Good enough is good enough for most things. Focus your efforts on what is truly most important in your life. You will have time to do this as you let go of perfect for everything else. Remember, good enough is good enough for most things. Save perfect for what really counts.

What Really Counts

I learn from my clients every day but one conversation in particular keeps coming back to me. My client, who had trouble holding on to jobs, related to me that he had been talking to his professionally successful older brother. Out of concern for my client's future, the successful brother asked him where he wanted to be in twenty years, most likely referring to my client's professional life. My client, who had been through a lot in the last couple of years and has done tremendous work on himself, answered, "To be happy."

What a perfect answer. To be happy is something worth trying to be perfect about but the rest of it...just forget perfect. Good enough is good enough.

Realize that what you find in this book is designed to help you toward a better life, a happier life. The goal is not to apply everything you find here perfectly. Use what you find in *Forget Perfect* in a way that works for you, with the knowledge that I am on this journey with you, not leading this journey but I am along for the ride.

Introduction

This book is designed to help you move your life forward while living with ADHD. It reflects what I have learned about ADHD from living with it and helping other people live with it in my work as an ADHD coach. The book reflects my experiences, observations, and ongoing training, which have been enriched by conversations with my clients, colleagues, and other specialists in the field of ADHD treatment. [1]

In it I suggest actions you can take to make your life easier and, I suspect, make the lives of those around you easier too. My hope is that reading and using this book will help you become more aware of some of the traps those of us with ADHD fall into and ways to release yourself from them so that you can put your energies into creating the life you want.

These traps include:

- *setting up systems for ourselves that are so complicated we don't end up using them*
- *going with our weaknesses rather than our strengths when deciding what career to pursue and other equally important decisions*
- *failing to do many things because we want to do them perfectly even though perfection is not possible*
- *spending a lot of time putting out fires rather than doing things we wish to do*

1. ADHD stands for Attention Deficit Hyperactivity Disorder. I use the term ADHD throughout the book because that is now what it is called whether or not you have hyperactivity.

I believe that there are ways of thinking, understanding, and being that help you avoid these pitfalls and act with confidence, that help you create the life you desire.

These include recognizing that:

- *You are not alone.*
- *Everybody has something they are dealing with.*
- *Striving for perfection is holding you back and is not necessary most of the time.*
- *You can live in a more anticipatory manner, dealing with what is and shaping what might be coming, even though it is hard for you.*
- *Following your intrinsic interests whenever possible will move you forward more quickly.*
- *Things can get better, and although you may fall back, you have the grit to get back up and move forward again.*
- *Getting back up and moving forward again and again is worth it because while perfection is highly overrated—life isn't.*

If you can realize that these are all true, then the obstacles ADHD presents are ones that you can overcome. I have seen it happen.

ADHD does in fact present you with particular challenges on your life's journey. This book supports your taking action and offers you practical approaches to meeting those challenges.

How to Use This Book

Read the book all the way through, a little at a time, or look at the topics in the table of contents and read what interests you. To make it easier to digest, the book includes tips, lists, and short essays so that you can flip through it or hunt out particular topics. At the end, I've included appendixes with additional information to help you on your journey in life with ADHD.

There is no one correct way to use this book. Above all use it in a way that works for you. I do encourage you to interact with it. Use the book as a learning tool, reference, awareness maker, jumping off point, or any other way you wish.

> ***Don't decide you have difficulty with something you don't just because it is mentioned in this book.***

We all are affected by ADHD in different ways. Know that not everything in the book will apply to everyone. Don't decide you have difficulty with something just because it is mentioned in the book. You know yourself best. Take what is helpful for you. You get to choose what you walk away with from reading this book. Don't force yourself to try and make what is not right for you work for you.

Some of the suggestions in the book may even contradict other suggestions. I say this because when you run across contradictory information I don't want you to think I am mix-ilated! (This is a "Wurf-word" that combines mixed-up and pixilated as in pixie dust. It means you're a little mixed up but in a quirky kind of way!) I am trying to provide for different types of people because different things work for different people. I hope most of the suggestions will work for you.

How This Book Is Organized

Much of the book is devoted to key areas of challenge for people affected by ADHD and reflects the persistent practical problems I have found come up repeatedly for my clients and myself, as someone affected by ADHD.

I hope to expand your vision for the kind of life you can have and to offer tools to help build that life. Chapter 1 helps you begin to look ahead, to start thinking about the shifts you need to make to move toward the life you desire. In it I introduce executive functions as providing the basis for an anticipatory approach to life.

Chapters 2-4 help you in moving toward some sense of control in the areas of task initiation, time management, and money management. These areas are challenging to everyone, but especially for those of us with ADHD. If you wish to create the life you want, you need to start here. These chapters cover the mundane, everyday stuff that requires attention to detail that many of us with ADHD don't like to deal with.

Chapters 5 and 6 provides help in setting up the habits and physical surroundings that give you a supportive structure and framework for your daily life.

The next two chapters, 7 and 8, help you interact with others in a more positive way, avoiding common pitfalls in communications and relationships.

Chapters 9 and 10 deal with navigating unemployment and the workplace, and emphasize finding work that leverages your strengths.

Chapter 11 provides quick hits on what I consider some of the most important messages in the book.

The Appendixes provide additional resources and more detailed guidance. To get updates to these resources, go to www.abigailwurf.com.

You can also sign up for my blog at http://abigailwurf.com/blog/

My hope is that you'll find the blog and this book of help on your journey.

Chapter One

Setting Your Destination

For those of us with ADHD it is harder to move into the future in an anticipatory fashion and shape what that future looks like. But you can do this, even if it's not second nature to you. This chapter will help you begin to move toward the life you desire as you start to identify what's important to you and become aware of the need to reject the negative attitudes that are so prevalent and so destructive for those of us with ADHD.

Executive Functions

What are executive functions? Executive functions are cognitive skills that help us interact in a meaningful way with the world by relating to actions or behaviors that take place in the future.

When working with my clients or explaining what executive functions are, I use these 12 categories or labels to break down executive functions. Here they are, in no particular order:

- *Planning*
- *Organizing*
- *Prioritizing*
- *Time Management*
- *Goal Setting*
- *Task Initiation* [2]
- *Focus*
- *Shift/Flexibility* [3]
- *Working Memory* [4]
- *Self-Inhibition* [5]
- *Emotional Regulation* [6]
- *Meta-cognition*

Everyone struggles with some or all of the executive functions, but for people affected by ADHD the difficulties are substantial and sustained—and the impact on their lives is significant. When I speak to clients about executive function problems, I talk about them in practical, concrete terms. For example, I might ask, "Do you feel you have more difficulty 'than the average bear' in managing long-term

2. Starting a task
3. Ability to move from one task or activity to another efficiently
4. How you use past memory along with current information to complete unusually complex tasks
5. Inhibiting behavior, usually impulsivity. The concept of thinking before you act.
6. Managing your emotions in situations in order to do what you set out to do

projects?" And then I follow up with:

- *Are you able to make a realistic timeline for how you will get the project done?*

- *Are you able to break the project down into smaller components and figure out the order you need to do them in?*

- *Do you have difficulty actually starting the project in time to get it done by its deadline?*

These three questions related to managing a long-term project help the client and me figure out if they have issues with executive functions like time management, task initiation, organization, prioritizing, and planning. (You'll notice that there is some overlap with executive functions. For example planning and prioritizing go hand-in-hand.)

The ability to access executive functions makes the difference in directing your life towards what you want to achieve based on your values or self-determined life mission. Many people affected by ADHD live reactively, from crisis to crisis. The phrase "full-catastrophe living" comes to mind. This phrase was coined by Jon Kabat-Zinn. Although he meant something different by the phrase, it conjures up an apt image for those of us with ADHD. I encourage you to move toward what the late Stephen R. Covey called a "purpose-driven life," what I call "purposeful living." That means living our lives striving for what we want rather than living reactively and dealing with what comes along because we think that is the best we can do.

As people with ADHD we need to exert effort to live purposefully. This effort involves developing systems and routines that help mitigate some of the havoc resulting from weak executive functions. This is what will move you substantially forward and give you the opportunities to create your purposeful life. That is what this book is about. It is also about helping you think about the possibilities for your life, what you are interested in, good at, and ultimately what you value in life. This self-knowledge is important for moving your life ahead—knowing where you are going.

Identifying Your Destination

If you are trying to move forward, you need to know the direction you want to go. For example, when you get in a car, on a bus, or in the subway, you have a destination in mind. Having that destination in mind is the stimulation that gets you activated to go somewhere. The same is true when trying to move forward in your life. You need to know what "forward" means to you. If you don't, you could end up going in circles or towards someone else's destination and not the destination meant for you.

How do you discover your destination? There are many ways to discover this. In the time management chapter, Chapter 3, I describe how to come up with your day-to-day priorities based on knowing your big "why's." Once you know that, you can determine your "wants" and "needs." Knowing your wants and needs as they relate to your big why's allows you to prioritize because you become clear on what actions align with your criteria and what actions do not. The result is a prioritized list of actions to take (and actions not to take), and what direction to go (and what directions not to go).

Establishing Your Intentions

You may have noticed that I haven't been using the word *goal* in discussing moving your life forward. Instead I focus on moving in a forward direction. That is because the word *goal* is a loaded one for people affected by ADHD. While I believe goals are necessary, I also think that initially it helps to think of your intentions. Goals are often part of a pass/fail paradigm that judges you on whether you either succeed (by reaching your goal) or fail (by falling short of it). This is not a good paradigm for people affected by ADHD, who have so often met failure. It is one reason many of those affected by ADHD don't like the word *goal*.

Intentions is a gentler word. It implies that moving toward your intentions is success, which it is. Here is another way to see this: instead of looking at your cup as being either full or empty (pass or fail), work on putting water in the cup little by little. Granted, some water will evaporate during the process but some water will also remain. As a result you are moving forward toward filling your cup. This is intentionality at work.

Setting Goals

Goals still have their place. Without setting some goals, we don't have to really hold ourselves accountable. Lacking goals diminishes our possibilities for success because our sense of what we are going after has become too hazy or watered down. What I advocate is learning to develop more specific goals with the understanding that change is constant and that our goals have to change to remain in alignment with changes going on within and without us.

People affected by ADHD do not do what I call "anticipatory living" very well, if at all. Anticipatory living is thinking past this moment to the next moment to the moment after that. It requires considering how what you are doing currently will shake out in the future and how what others are doing will affect you in the future. Dr. Ned Hallowell says for people with ADHD there is "now" and "not now." We have to force ourselves to anticipate the "what is to come."

Making goals can help because it keeps us looking toward the future and gives us a toehold of sorts for tracking what is going on around us and what we need to start thinking about for the future.

In 1999, I had disastrous back surgery that ended up making me worse, not better. As a result I decided to go to graduate school in dance and education. I had always enjoyed teaching dance, dance choreography, and dance history.

After I finished my master's, I still applied and got into the doctoral program. But I hadn't reflected upon what being in a doctoral program meant in terms of workload and expectations. A month and a half in, it was clear that I had made a mistake. I didn't even know what I would have done with the degree. I wasn't thinking far enough in advance, nor was I anticipating the challenges ahead of me.

That was a little over fifteen years ago, and I have moved on with my life and have set goals, but, until recently, never concrete ones. The goals were always in my mind and therefore easily dismissed because they were not written down or publicly proclaimed.

To commit to a goal it is necessary to write it down and declare yourself—otherwise it is not really real. It is easier now for me to set specific goals because I understand executive function skills. Goal setting is about making a plan. And making a plan is about:

- *prioritizing what you want*
- *figuring out how to get it*
- *determining the order of the steps you need to take*
- *identifying the materials or support you will need*
- *getting started and sustaining action*
- *staying on task*
- *recalibrating when things don't go as you thought they would*
- *managing yourself during the process and anyone else you need to work with or who crosses your path*
- *finally, keeping on schedule*

If you look back to the executive function list, that pretty well covers them all.

ADHD and Resistance to Goal Setting

Many of us have difficulty setting goals for ourselves. We may vaguely say we want to get more done or do better at our career but these are not motivating goals. To be motivating, goals must be specific and realistic. If we feel that we are pursuing an important goal that we set, it helps in getting what we need to get done, especially professionally.

Many of us don't like to be pinned down by specifics. Setting a specific goal and writing it down can be scary. It means that failure is possible. Nonetheless, it is important to have specific goals if you want to achieve forward progress in your life.

Creating Global Goals and Identifying Your Roles

When you set specific goals, you want to base them on your global goals, which are by nature long-term. Your intermediate and short-term goals will support your global goals. Know that your goals will shift as you move forward in your life because change is inevitable. In order to live purposefully, with every change you must be able to adjust, re-creating your goals as you move forward. Here is one approach to getting a sense of your global goals:

1. Figure out what your real mission is in life. You can do this by writing a mission statement like organizations do. I suggest thinking in terms of one's big "why's," as in "Why am I here? What am I here to do?" Your answer can be on a global scale, such as wanting every child to have an education, on a local level, such as wanting to rid your community of gang-related violence, or on a personal level, such as making sure your children have the best launch into adulthood you can provide.

   Almost everyone has more than one "why." For me, much of my big "why" is helping people affected by ADHD move their lives forward and offering both paid services and free services to support that. Another "why" is to be financially solvent so I am not a burden to my family or society.

2. Once you know your why's you can figure out your roles in life. My roles regarding ADHD include coach, consultant, writer, speaker, and educator. My roles as a business owner include employer, program developer, and marketer. At a personal level there are my roles as a daughter, sister, aunt, and friend. An important role not to forget is myself as an individual. One of my why's is individual growth.

Research has shown that the average person cannot manage more than seven roles. I suggest trying to keep it down to five. One of the ways I do that is by making my roles more general.

My Roles (in no particular order):

Family Member and Friend – daughter/sister/aunt/friend

Business Owner – visionary, coach, consultant, employer, etc.

Volunteer – local public radio station, ADHD organization

Individual – personal growth, actions align with values, citizen, health

Sharpening the Saw [7] *– improving my skills and capacities in all my roles*

7. Stephen Covey tells a story called Sharpening the Saw as a metaphor for the importance of self-renewal and self-improvement. For Covey that includes working on our nature, which he defines as a combination of the "physical, spiritual, mental and social/emotional (*Seven Habits of Highly Effective People*, p. 288).

A Method for Finding Out Your Why's

If you get stuck trying to figure out your goals, first look at your roles and then look at your "why's." What are your roles? What is your goal or "why" for each role you have in your life?

Use Your Why's to Prioritize

Once you know your why's it is easier to prioritize. If you have difficulties with time management it is likely you are unrealistic as to what you can accomplish in a day or a week. This means that some things have to go. Prioritizing helps you decide what goes.

> ***Needs are things you can't live without.***
>
> ***Wants are things you would really like but can live without.***
>
> ***Your WHYs will help you sort this out.***

Look at your why's and from those figure out what your values are. Then from your values figure out your needs and your wants. Needs are things you can't live without and wants are things you would really like but can live without. Wants and needs can change places. If you live in a city with lots of public transportation, a car is a want—not a need. If you live in a rural area where there is no public transportation and the closest job is miles away, as is the grocery store, then a car can become a need. You will find more on this in Chapter 3, Time Management (Managing Actions).

What does all this have to do with ADHD and forgetting perfect? A lot. This focuses you on what you need to do, what you want to do, and what you can do—not what you think you should do.

Clearing Out Negativity

To develop the life we want we also need to be clear about things that get in our way. For those of us affected by ADHD, we encounter in ourselves many and varied forms of negativity and self-destructive behavior.

I have never met a person affected by ADHD who wasn't tied down and held back in some fashion by judging themselves negatively, dwelling in what I call the "Land of Shoulding: I should have done that, I should have done this." This is not fun territory to inhabit, and while dwelling there you tend to waste time trying to figure out what you assume others are thinking about you.

Above all, this gets in the way of moving forward toward your goals. Just as you can hold yourself back by poor emotional regulation and self-inhibition (executive functions), you can move yourself forward with good emotional regulation and self-inhibition. A good place to start is by taking on any and all negativity in yourself.

Getting Clear through the Body

How do you get clear on what's important to you? What your roles are? We have it right in our grasp. According to Erick Hawkins, "The body is a clear place." Erick Hawkins was one of the founders of American modern dance and he believed that in order to move you had to let go of all affectations and tensions. Movement came from a centered place and a clear body. As he said, "tense muscles cannot feel," meaning if you moved with tense muscles you were not free to really feel what your body was supposed to feel to create the true movement.

When I start thinking about how I could make my body, especially my mind, "a clear place," just as tense muscles are freed to move when they are relaxed, it became easier to just do what I needed to do. Letting go of all the judgmental junk, even for a half hour, was a half hour of peace and improved productivity. And this is a hell of an easier way to live. Furthermore, my resistance to pinning down my goals and making plans has diminished somewhat.

To achieve your goals you need to stop dwelling on or, as a few us do, luxuriating, in all the failure, could have beens, never wills, and negative assumptions. Like most familiar territory it is hard to leave. It appears to be a place of safety because we know the terrain so well, but this familiarity is holding you back. Start now. Begin making changes even before you believe you will move forward. Just take some of the tips and suggestions in this book and do them. Just do.

What does all this have to do with executive functions and forgetting perfect?

- *If you want to go anywhere or achieve anything it is your executive functions that will get you there.*
- *If you are waiting for the perfect moment to get a move on it, you will never move on it.*
- *Some of us tend to hold ourselves back by setting no goals or intentions because we think it is safer not to.*

But not doing anything is what's not safe. And more to the point, don't all of us want a better life, based on what's important to us?

Forget Perfect

Strengthening your executive functions will help you live in an anticipatory manner.

Consider setting your intentions before you set goals.

Exert the effort it takes to live purposefully.

Figuring out your "why's" and your roles in life will help you set priorities.

Don't wait to believe you can change; start making changes now.

Chapter Two

Starting and Completing Tasks

There are all kinds of reasons we don't get stuff done. We may have problems starting on a task or getting stuck in the middle of it. We may have problems sticking to the task and completing it. Maybe we're overwhelmed, fearful that we can't do it, or just bored. Maybe we've done some of the work—even a lot of work—but we can't see a path to getting to the end. We may get bogged down in focusing on how long we can work on the task rather than how long we should work on it. That's what this chapter is about. Oh, and it's also about the P-word... procrastination. (See, I even put that off too, until the last part of this paragraph!)

Overcome Overwhelm

I should be preparing for a speech I need to give tonight. The speech is not even finished!

It is now 11am. I got myself up at 7am to get to work on it. I ate and promptly went back to bed. Got up again around 8:30am, ate some more, looked at my emails, made a call and went back to bed again! Got back up at 10:30am, looked at emails, Amazon, and now I am writing this!

You may be familiar with this story. Something big and important has to get done and you just can't get yourself to work on it.

Part of the problem is that I am overwhelmed. After I finish the speech I have to start on two proposals that are due in two days. Once I start working, the work isn't going to stop for a while. I am thinking about all that needs to get done. I am also a little resentful of all the work even though it is all my doing.

To overcome feeling overwhelmed, I know that I need to clear my mind. Here are a few ways I've learned to do this.

Have Someone Else Hold Your Worries

Tell someone else your worries and concerns. While that other person "holds" those worries for you, take the steps you need to get going. It helps clear my mind to just remind myself that my friend Betty is holding that other stuff for me right now. My job is simply to get to work and accomplish my task. I will let her know that she may be hearing from me again if I need more worries to be held or need a boost.

My one caveat with this approach is to make sure that you pick the right person to hold your worries, someone who will truly support you and will not hold it over you that she or he has done this big favor.

Know That It's Not As Bad As You Think

Sometimes you're putting off what you need to do because you think you can't do it or believe it's too hard for you. Try just getting down to it. Do the work and ask for help if you need to. You may well find that it wasn't nearly as bad—either as hard or as long a task—as you thought it would be. Your fear that you can't do it may really be about your fear of how big you think the project will be.

I am always surprised that when I actually sit down to do whatever I've put off, it's really not as hard as I thought it would be. My mind had created many more obstacles than were there. Often I find out that the hand wringing I went through was unnecessary and unwarranted. The irony here is that usually once you simply take action, virtually any action related to the project or task, you discover not only that your fears were unwarranted but also that it kind of feels good and empowering to be getting the project or task done. There is a sense of "kicking butt and taking names."

So how does this work? Why do we do this to ourselves? How do we get into this state of fear? This has nothing to do with how long something took compared to how long I thought it would take, but with fear of my own ability to be able to do the task—or, more precisely, my fear of not being able to do the task perfectly.

It's this fear that stopped me. If I somehow believed that someone else were doing this task, they would do it the right way, and if I only knew for sure that right way.... Then once you actually do that thing, you realize it can no longer be perfect. That perfect thing you imagine is no longer possible. In this moment is liberation, for you have given up the perfect for doing the work and getting it the done.

I tend to get behind in my bookkeeping. By December I was way behind. I hadn't done anything since May! I looked at the mess of papers I had and didn't know how to begin. So I phoned a friend. She suggested I start by sorting the papers by month. I did that. Then I was confused about what to do next. "Don't you usually input the expenses by month in a chronological order?" she asked. Yes, but I told her it was more difficult than that. "Why don't you just try?" she asked. Reluctantly I did, and I started getting it done, month by month.

Unfortunately I have to admit that occasionally it is also about simply not wanting to do the task and, truth be told, maybe deep down inside I am hoping if I sound confused enough the other person will either help me or do the task for me. This is not an attractive action or manipulation, whether conscious or not. In cases like this it is best to just be vigilant and catch yourself when you realize you are simply trying to fob off the task onto someone else. You will be stronger for it and wiser for doing it.

Figure Out How Long to Spend on a Task

Thinking about how long you *can* work on a task instead of how long you *should* work on it is a difficult thing for many people affected by ADHD.

For people who have trouble sticking to tasks and completing tasks, I find it ironic that we often work too hard and long on many tasks, more so than other people. I believe that this is because we don't pre-think the value of a task. To put it in business terms, if someone asks you to write an article about penguins and is willing to pay you $50, most people would spend what they deemed was a fair trade of their time for the $50. If instead you were offered $5,000 to write an article about penguins, the amount of time most people would put into the project would increase commensurate to the money they are being paid. What many of us do instead is put in the same amount of time and effort regardless of how much we are being paid or how important the project or task is in the bigger scheme of things.

For things that are of little value or importance, we should put little time and effort into them, and the corollary is true. For things that are of great value or importance, a great amount of time and effort should be exerted. This seems obvious on the surface but, time and time again, I find my clients and me spending too much time on the little things and not enough time on the big things that can affect our future.

Getting Started

For those of us affected by ADHD, getting started is a major obstacle to getting tasks done. When we're anxious or fearful that we can't do the task in front of us, we may be tied up thinking that there's a perfect way to do the task. Once we start, we realize it no longer has the possibility of being perfect or that it is unlikely we will produce something perfect.

Take One Baby Step at a Time

When you find you're procrastinating, start with the three smallest baby tasks you can do and then take a break. Repeat and eventually you will continue to work, forgetting that you were only going to take three baby steps.

Baby steps are really little tasks that you can make yourself do:

- *sitting down at your desk,*
- *finding your pen, and*
- *getting a piece of paper for a to do list.*

After a break, you may want to title that page "To do." That counts as a step.

Keeping these first tasks small creates less resistance and makes them feel doable.

Start in the Middle—or Skipping the Crawl

When I was two years old I hadn't crawled, much less stood up or walked. I sat there, not moving around, and was carried from place to place. That summer my family rented a beach house that had open stairs. They brought no gates with them because my brother was five and was already a good walker.

Once we got to the beach house I immediately stood up and started to toddle around. No crawling for me. Just straight to the point. With no gates to prevent me from trying the open stairs it was quite dangerous. Needless to say, we ended that vacation early and went home where things could be controlled better.

Skipping the crawl is about skipping the beginning and starting in the middle.

We usually think we need to start at the beginning and often we are not sure how to do that. Don't let that stop you. Just plow ahead and start somewhere else. Then move to the next step. If you can't do that, then go to the next step until you find something you can do. In many situations you might have to go back and fill in whatever you left blank.

Not sure how to start at the beginning? Don't let that stop you. Just move to the next step until you find something you can do.

Worried you might go in a wrong direction this way? That is okay. Even though you have to redo some things, you have at least started. Task initiated! Sometimes you don't know how to start at the beginning. If that's the case, skip it! You will still find success. I did. I became a professional dancer—despite being late to walking.

Get Mad

Sometimes the feeling of being overwhelmed ties you up inside. You are frustrated, resentful, and want to quit, but that thing still has to get done. This may be the time to get your mad on. Get mad, angry, and hostile. Then rage, be unreasonable, obnoxious, and bull-headed. Say I will not be defeated. By this time every atom within you is perched on edge, ready to fight the fight. All else fades to black as you plunge into what has got to get done.

Stay mad, feed the anger, luxuriate in it. It is power. Screw all the forces pushing against you, getting in your way. Fade everything into a blackness that surrounds you so you can keep everyone and everything out and do what must be done.

Then when you are done, breathe. Release the anger. It might already be gone since you finished your task or project.

Note: You have to have the right personality to make this work. Use this technique sparingly as it can be detrimental to people and objects nearby.

Get Clear by Making a Plan

You have a project due tomorrow, and instead of working on it you are writing a Facebook entry (or, fill in the blank with your favorite p-activity, as in procrastination). You aren't quite sure how to proceed. Not knowing how to proceed is getting in the way and causing procrastination. The lack of a clear next step is causing you to just avoid settling down to work at all.

The usual advice would be to break down the project into smaller pieces to make it more approachable and then start piece by piece. But what if you can't see how to break it down into pieces? What if you have done all the research but you don't know how to put all the random information into a logical order? There are many possible approaches to take at this point.

- *Talk to a friend or family member.* Describe the project and see if that person has any ideas. If it's a research project, then describe your research. How did you end up describing it to them? Where did you begin, etc
- *Dictate into the computer.* Most computers have voice recognition software that you can dictate your ideas into the computer and then sort through them later.
- *The index card method.* Brainstorm the major topics and write down one idea per card. Then start playing around with different orders for the cards until you find what flows and what to eliminate (also important).
- *Brain dump.* Free write everything you know on the topic, then move the information around into some cohesive form. While brain dumping, don't think about form at all. Just let your ideas flow.
- *Outline the information.* Using your index card deck (see above) create a written outline based on that information.
- *Mind map the information.* Mind mapping is when you put the main topic in the center of a page and then draw lines out from the center to related topics. Then you draw lines out from those topics to sub topics, etc. Mind

mapping gives a visual way to organize. (For a list of mind mapping apps, see Appendix E: Information Management)

These are just some ideas to help get clear and start making a plan. The next steps are even harder for us: executing the plan. Yet these approaches work: index cards followed by creating an outline is how this book came into being.

Identify the Steps You Need to Take and Execute Your Plan

To finish your task or project you need to have a plan and then make sure to execute it relentlessly—despite your desire to throw it overboard.

Step 1: Plan...but *planning is worthless* (or so we think)! *A complete exercise in futility* (or so we believe)! Why? Because we don't do Step 2. Step 2 is harder so we tend to shy away from it.

Step 2: Implement the plan consistently! That means sticking to it each and every day, and not just when we feel like it. This step is incredibly hard for people like us.

To succeed at Step 2, be very clear about your goals and very specific about each step you need to take to achieve them. That way you will not have to tease out what step you need to take each day. If you have a strong, specific plan your next step will be clear.

Step 3: Continue to stick with the plan. Be a slave to it. This will be hard. We like to chase shimmery new objects and ideas, not a stale old plan. We also tend to go off on tangents.

Step 4: If help is offered, make sure that it's from someone you trust and would be comfortable to reciprocate with another favor.

Step 5: Get back to the plan. Don't get distracted from your bigger priorities.

Step 6: Never lose sight on the why—why you are doing what you are doing. Remind yourself each day of your why to stay motivated.

Step 7: Stick to the plan. Don't overdo it one day because you feel like you are on a roll and getting a lot of stuff done. If you overdo on one day, you won't want to work the next day due to burn out, and then once you've skipped a day you will have lost momentum. It will be difficult to restart your plan. It may even stop you from continuing to follow your plan at all.

This step-by-step process can make it easier to get things done, especially if you give yourself time to carry it out. But for those of us with ADHD, we often use time differently—to force the issue so that we have to act. This doesn't always work, and we can find ourselves in denial about the task and a looming deadline.

When Pressure Doesn't Help You Get Things Done

That nth moment, when it is now or never, usually activates us to start. But sometimes the opposite happens and the pressure to get something done stalls us out.

Right before the nth moment is a lull when we are either in a state of shock or detached from reality. This is a place we are liable to get stuck in. It is as if there is *no* pressure. The looming event is not an immediate reality. You feel as if you have all the time in the world. Why not take a nap!

This is a sign of avoidance and fear. Fear creates a situation of disbelief—disbelief that you really *are* in trouble and need to get to work.

How do you shake out of it before it is too late? You'll have to find out what works for you. Here are some ideas to try out.

- *Make a list of what has to happen by what time. Assign realistic time increments for each action.*
- *Sit quietly to calm down and come to a state of acceptance that there is only so much time. Then ask yourself, What can I realistically get done in that time?*
- *Go to a friend, parent, colleague, or coach and ask for some help getting back on track.*
- *Write about it in a public forum so that you remember that you know what to do and it is time to activate (as we say in ADHD parlance).*
- *Ask yourself, What would I tell a friend to do? Then take your own advice and do that!*

These techniques can help when you're overwhelmed or fearful, but what if you plain just don't want to do the work? What then?

Getting Things Done That You Don't Want to do

Every adult, with ADHD or not, finds themselves with things they just don't want to do staring them in the face. If you are affected by ADHD, this poses more of a challenge. You get overwhelmed, or feel unmotivated, or simply believe you just aren't up to the task. What do you do then?

I was doing what many people with ADHD hate to do: making phone calls. And I was making multiple phone calls to three different businesses trying to get information about vacation rentals. It involved so many details, including searching and viewing the different properties on the web while asking numerous questions and keeping straight which house had what (price, number of bedrooms and baths, number of stairs, dates of availability, Internet, washer/dryer, etc.) and where it was located.

Furthermore, I was with someone who was making comments and asking questions while I was on the phone with the different realtors. My attention was flying—screen, phone, other person, my brain, notes, ahhhhh!

I could have gotten really agitated, but no one was at fault. Things were just happening all at once, which can be hard to manage. My ingrained response is to push back or get impatient or irritated. I decided I wasn't going to let that happen, even though I felt like letting off a little steam. Instead I decided to make the process kind of...well, adventure would be too strong a word, but let's say a brain expedition in rugged territory.

It became like an obstacle course I had to get through, except instead of challenging my body, it was challenging my mind not to lose my cool.

Sometimes when we have to do things we don't like or that are not our strongest skill set, approaching it as a challenge can ease some of the frustration and emotional exertion and allows us to just get it done. I felt tired but good after the 3 hours—yes, *3 hours*—it took to resolve the issue. I stuck with it, kept my cool, and achieved a good result.

Stop Expecting to Enjoy

I made a major breakthrough one week. I gave up!

I was doing twice a week Pilates workouts at a studio. I had scheduled appointments with an individual instructor. I had pre-paid for the lessons. As a result, I was successful at arriving at the appointments and doing the workouts.

But then I realized that six months of appointments would more than pay for the equipment I needed to do the exact same workout at home. So I decided to buy the equipment and work out at home. No more commute or scheduling issues. I'd save time and money. I'd even increase my practice to three times a week.[8]

Much easier, right?

Wrong! My first mistake was to up the number of times I worked out a week. I had been going twice a week with support, now I was planning to do it on my own and do it three times a week. My second mistake was assuming I would feel the same pull to work out that I did when I met with my instructor. Instead I found that I didn't feel the pull to work out at home.

Within weeks I was facing failure. I found I wasn't initiating the workouts. I would go into the room to exercise, and then begin to think of why I didn't want to, and then I wouldn't exercise. Some of reasons I would not work out were crazy and unreasonable:

8. Important: If you are starting a workout routine, check with your doctor and get some help to be sure you are doing things correctly. Doing exercises incorrectly can cause injuries. Especially if you use equipment, make sure to have someone help you to use it efficiently and safely. The only reason I purchased the Pilates equipment is because I have gone through the Pilates Certificate Teacher Training Program.

It would mean another shower

It was too early in the morning and would disturb my neighbors

It was too late in the evening and would disturb my neighbors

It was too much effort to put on my workout clothes

It would add to the amount of laundry that would need to be done

There wasn't enough time for a full workout

I was not in the mood to sweat

I would have to wipe down the equipment after use whereas now it was clean

(The laundry excuse was particularly ridiculous because I don't even do my own laundry!)

As is true for many things, once I got started working out it wasn't so bad. Sometimes, I even enjoyed myself. But going from thinking I should exercise to actually initiating the activity, an executive function, stymied me. I found this extremely frustrating because even as I chose not to work out, I remembered I found the activity was fun once I got started.

To take this on, the first thing I did was *lower my expectations*. I reduced the number of workouts from three to two times a week. That took a lot of stress off me. With one less failure a week I could make my goal to increase to three times a week once I got twice a week down pat.

Then the real breakthrough occurred. *I stopped expecting to enjoy this.* I had been waiting for the pull, the desire to do the workout, but the truth is that I don't like exercising. So why was I expecting to want to do something I didn't like doing?

I find brushing my teeth and taking a shower really boring, but I do it anyway because of the ramifications if I don't. What were the ramifications if I didn't exercise? I would get weaker, fatter, lose stamina, become less healthy and probably less attractive. I realized that wanting to do something is "lousy criteria" for getting something as important as exercise done.

Letting go of the idea and the expectation of joy or desire freed me up to just do it. It is Friday, I exercise on Fridays. It is Saturday, I don't exercise on Saturdays. Simple, I pick my days and just like I shower, I exercise.

This has taken an awful lot of stress off me. Exercising seems more automatic and a part of what I do to live. I don't have those internal arguments every day about whether I will or will not do it. It is not up for discussion anymore. The workout is more rote.

If I do feel I need to develop some support system, I can work with my instructor once a month for a tune-up to make sure I am doing things correctly and advancing properly. This will encourage me to work out during the week so there is improvement between the monthly sessions with her.

Dealing with Boredom

I don't have those internal arguments every day about whether I will or will not do it. It is not up for discussion anymore.

Someone with ADHD is more likely to get a task done if it is intrinsically of interest to them. This doesn't mean they may not still struggle with it, just that they are more likely to do it. Conversely, if you're not interested in the task, you're likely to avoid it and struggle with completing it. If you're finding this to be true for you, reread Stop Expecting to Enjoy!

What is it that you want to incorporate in your life and forget about whether you want to do it or whether you enjoy it? Think about how you can make it a part of your routine and stop leaving it up to daily internal discussions as to whether or not you are going to follow through. This may be a new way for you to approach getting things done.

To Keep Up the Momentum, Stop in the Middle

What if you've started on a task or project, but then fear that you'll lose momentum and languish?

When you are working on a long project, leave in the middle of a thought. If you have to take a break or you no longer can work on the project that day, do not wait to stop at a logical endpoint. Otherwise, when you come back to the project, you won't know what you need to do to move forward and it is hard to start working again.

It is as though you were on a sailboat and it has become becalmed, which means there is no wind and the water is smooth. The sailboat is as still as anything can be when floating on water. Unless you have a motor on the sailboat, you simply have to wait until the wind picks up again or get a tow from a motorboat. There is really nothing you can do on your own.

That is why, when you take a break or finish for the day, leave in the middle of an idea or in the middle of an action. Let's take a writing project, for example. Don't finish the section or the sentence. Leave in the middle of it because when you come back there will be some action ready and waiting for you to take. You can then pick up again by finishing the sentence or finishing the idea in the section. By starting where you know what to do, you build up the momentum that helps you go on to the next idea and the next action.

Working this way you will never have to go back to a project that is at a dead stop. Instead it's as though there is an arrow pointing you in the right direction when you decide to restart the project.

I would also suggest another arrow: an arrow that points to the word *celebrate*.

Celebrate!

An important component of getting projects done is celebrating your victories! Don't dwell on whether you got the work done in exactly the fashion you planned. The most important thing is that you got it done. You persisted.

> ***In a curious way, ask yourself: What got in my way of getting the project done in a timely manner? What can I learn from that experience for the future?***

People affected by ADHD tend to focus on what didn't work rather on what did. We always look for reasons to judge ourselves. And that judgment is almost always negative.

Yeah, I got it done, but I didn't get it done by the time I had planned. Stop! You got it done, that is the important part. When you are in a good place, you may want to reflect back, in a curious manner not negative one:

- *What got in my way of getting the project done in a timely manner?*
- *What can I learn from that experience for the future?*
- *What is something I could do pro-actively before the next project?*

Ask people who you know are good planners or project managers how they get stuff done. Choose to try something you think might work for you the next time. Look at each new plan or project as an experiment in trying out new approaches to see if they will work for you. Again, be curious in your approach to trying something new, not judging your potential success or failure before you try.

Nothing is all good or bad, black or white. You can learn from each opportunity rather than using it to judge yourself. In any situation you can find something to celebrate or to judge. The choice is yours.

Forget Perfect

Clear your mind by telling your worries to someone you trust.

Make a plan for finishing up the task or project and then stick to the plan. This way you're clear about the actions you need to take.

Get your momentum going by starting with the smallest steps you can imagine.

If you're mad, frustrated, whatever you're feeling, express it (safely) and let it go. Then get down to work and get 'er done!

When you finish a task, celebrate!

Chapter Three

Time Management (Managing Your Actions)

Time management is a lie. Time is finite. You can't bend it, stretch it, or manipulate it. But while you can't manage time, you can manage your actions. If you consider and manage these actions in a way that supports your values and goals, you have the best chance of moving life forward in the direction you choose. In this chapter I point out some things that get in the way of managing actions and present techniques for working with them. Once you've read some of the pitfalls I've fallen into, you may feel that your situation is not hopeless at all!

For those of us with ADHD, it is especially important to manage and direct our actions. We tend to get pulled in many directions, depending on what's in front of us. Unless we find a way to overcome this tendency, we're unlikely to be able to live the life we want.

Let Your Values Determine Your Actions

How can we start to manage our actions? There are only so many actions you can take in a day, so many possibilities for that day. When you align your actions with your values, you are only acting on what is important to you and to the people you care about. This requires going through a process of first figuring out your values—identifying what's important to you—and figuring out your needs and your wants.

You need to know what your big WHYs are. Why are you here? What is the reason for your existence? What were you put here to do? How can you serve others while on the planet? You can tie religion into this exploration or not. The point is that in order to live a good life, you need a reason to move forward. Your reason(s) are your WHY and answering the "why" question helps you figure out your values. Your answers will be different than others', and they will also depend on the stage of life you are in.

What does this have to do with time management? You can use all this information as a filter to help you decide what actions are imperative, preferred, unnecessary, or damaging to you. Knowing this helps you manage your actions, which in turn determines how you use your time. Remember: it is not time you are managing. You are managing your actions so that they (and you) stay in alignment with your big WHYs and your values. In doing so, you are living a powerfully considered life.

Knowing your big WHYs is not a one-time thing. You must continue to examine them over the course of your lifetime because with major life changes, your values can change. For example, in the past you may not have valued having children. Now you want to have them.

Distinguish Between Needs and Wants

In addition to identifying your values, it's important to distinguish between your needs and your wants.

Needs are those things that are necessary for you to live. Wants are those things that you desire but could survive without. Nothing says you can't have your wants, but if they are taking precedence over meeting your needs, you'll want to put your needs first.

For example, we could live without a roof over our heads but most people have a need to have some sort of home. Another need is food because we cannot survive without sustenance. Wants are things we can live without. TV is a want. Shocking as this may be for some of you, a smartphone is a want.

Wants and needs change as times change. For example, it is getting to a point where most of us need some sort of connection to the Internet to take care of the obligations of modern day living. Fifteen years ago, the Internet was more a want than a need.

It is important to distinguish between needs and wants because before you try to address your wants, you need to fulfill or be working towards fulfilling your needs. That is because in your life a want might be getting in the way of, or taking priority over, a need. Again, it's important to note that needs and wants are not static. They shift as your values and your life situation shifts, and they vary from person to person.

For example, say you do not live near public transportation and your car is in need of repair. One of your values is keeping a roof over your family's head and food on the table. If you can't get to work, you may lose your job and the only employer is 15 miles away. In this case, you car is not a want but a need and therefore must be fixed. But if instead of saving money to repair your car, you keep spending money, ordering wants over the Internet. You have forgotten that you need to focus meeting your needs first.

I recommend you put your exact situation down on paper. That makes it more real and more actionable.

Using Your Values, Wants, and Needs to Guide Your Actions

Here is a simplified process based on what I take people through in one of my seminars

- *Make a list of all your current time management difficulties. These might include getting to work, cleaning your home, calling your Mom, etc.*
- *Number the items based on the biggest difficulty down to the smallest difficulty.*
- *Make a short list of your whys.*
- *Make a short list of your main values.*
- *Create two columns side by side: one "needs" and the other "wants."*
- *Distribute your time management items into the appropriate column.*
- *List "needs" in order of descending importance (from most to least important).*
- *Take your organizer or planning calendar and schedule your week, based on filling in the needs in order of the list. When your time is filled, those are the needs that you can accomplish.*

Manage Your Actions by Using an Organizer or Planning Calendar

Usually those of us with ADHD are not good at sensing the passage of time, estimating time, and budgeting time. For that reason we have difficulty planning and managing our actions. One of the most important tools we can use to help us manage our actions is an organizer or planning calendar.

Whether what you use is electronic or paper, it doesn't matter. The most important thing is that you consistently use the tool you choose to direct your actions toward your goals.

I have developed the habit of looking at my calendar when I get up in the morning, at lunch when I take a break, before or after dinner, and then at bedtime.

Many people use their phone because it's small, it can fit in a pocket or purse, and they carry it with them most of the time. These computer planner calendars often are integrated with a to do list, which helps to focus on tasks while scheduling them. If the to do list is separate it is more likely that important things don't get done.

I am one of those ADHD people who is terrible with time. I have no sense of time passing or of how long different tasks take me. I even forget appointments. For that reason, my organizer has become my lifeline. I use a paper organizer because there's no screen to go black (like the cell phone, tablet, or computer). I keep my organizer open to the current week, and it sits right next to me at all times while I am working. I have also developed the habit of looking at it when I get up in the morning, when I take a break, before for lunch, after dinner, and then at bedtime to prepare for the next day.

The organizer I use is called the Planner Pad® organizer (I do not get any money by recommending this product). It helps me manage my time more effectively and keeps my plan of action visible at all times. The Planner Pad organizer is a 3-tier funnel system that helps me with planning. I start with listing tasks, the things I want to get done in the different areas of my life. Then I prioritize these tasks, and finally I schedule them.

The organizer is designed so that you can see one whole week at a time. When open, you see 8 columns across the two pages: seven columns for each day of the week and an eighth column with room to make notes, track expenses, and view the prior and following months. There are three tiers in the weekly section: from the top, the first tier is where you organize tasks into categories that need to be done in the current week or in future weeks, the middle tier is where you prioritize your tasks by day, and the third tier is where you schedule and block out time to complete tasks.

In the first tier you organize your tasks into categories. My categories are marketing, client services, financial, and administrative. I also have a column for my volunteer work. Another column is labeled *personal,* for anything I need to do that's not related to my coaching business. There's a seventh column in that row, which you can use for another category.

After I categorize my tasks, I use the second tier to prioritize them by the day of the week I want to get them done. Finally I schedule tasks in the bottom section, the appointment book section. Whatever tasks I don't schedule, I still have visibility on so that I can get those tasks done as I have time and if I choose to do them.

(The website for Planner Pads® is *www.plannerpads.com*. Be sure to order their Insta Pockets for the front and back of your calendar. This will insure that you have places to stick important notes, prescriptions, and any other important loose pieces of paper you might need with you.)

Know Your Schedule and Your Tasks

Whatever organizer or planning calendar you use, it is important to know you have activities for each day of the week. With the Planner Pad® organizer, you can see the week of scheduled activities. This organizer allows you to see when and where you will get things done and the funneling process helps you break everything down into manageable chunks and schedule them.

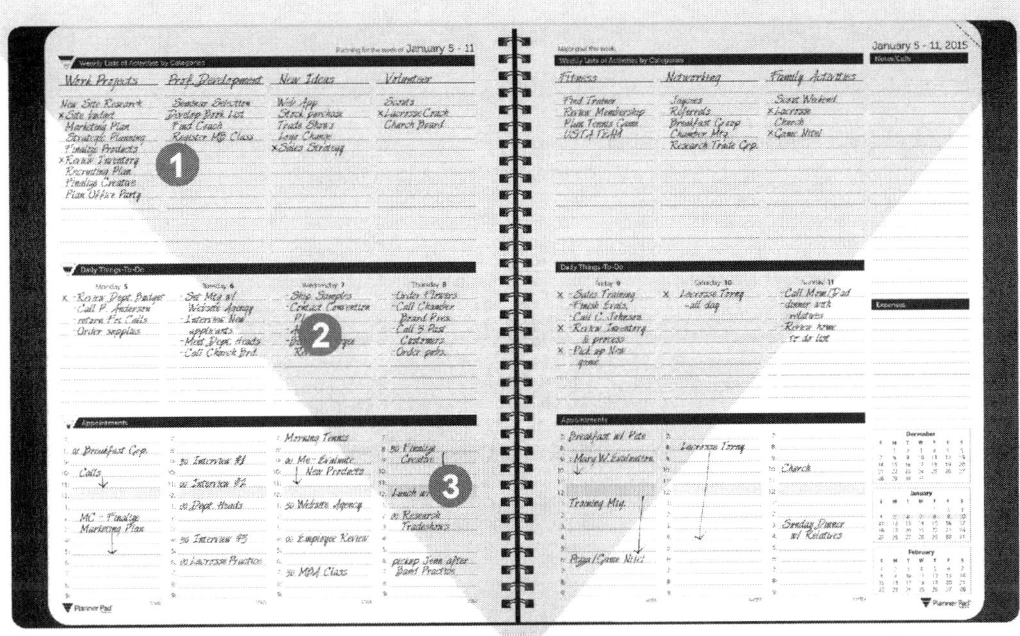

Make Your Organizer or Planning Calendar Your Constant Companion

Carry your organizer or planner with you at all times. By doing this, you're less likely to forget tasks and appointments. Furthermore, no matter where you are you can record important information and know where to retrieve it. You can make appointments on the spot and not have to call someone back once you check your calendar. Finally after finishing tasks, phone calls, or appointments, you can record them in your organizer or planning calendar, writing any important details you think you might forget.

Track Past, Present, and Future

Your organizer or planning calendar can also serve as a record of the past that you can refer to in the future. For example, if you put money in a CD, noting when you do that can help you track when it is up for renewal. I find it especially helpful to plug in names and addresses related to appointments I have. I will also note anything I might want to remember about that appointment, such as how to get there or an assistant's name or the name of the great restaurant I went to. When I am trying to remember this information at a later date, I can usually think of approximately when I last dealt with that person or place and know where to find the information I am looking for.

Write down successes in your calendar. When you're feeling frustrated or low, they will remind you of your strengths and can do ability.

If I have a doctor's appointment and the doctor orders a test, I mark this in my book so I know to follow up on the results. I also then have a record of when the test was administered, what the test was for, and who administered it. Finally, as we all know, tax time comes every year. If you keep detailed notes and follow up information in your calendar it can be very helpful in reconstructing last year's financial life.

Note Your Successes

No doubt you will run into frustrations as those of us affected with ADHD work with managing our actions. For that reason, be especially vigilant about writing down successes in your organizer or appointment book. When you're feeling frustrated or low, reviewing your achievements will help remind you of your strengths and "can do" ability.

Dealing with Being Late, Overcommitting, and Other ADHD Time Issues

Time creates difficulty for those of us affected by ADHD, and managing our actions is something that's hard for us to do. Okay, that's the bad news. The good news is that there are ways to work out our situations.

Be Careful of Becoming a Pleaser

We are poor estimators of time and in an effort to please people, we often make promises we can't possibly keep given the time we have, even if we could fly! As a result we are often late. This pleases no one. Often to try and make the situation better or to make up for being late, we promise more the next time without considering what our schedules demand of us, and so we disappoint again. This becomes a pattern. As a result, we are thought of as being unreliable.

Before you say *yes* to please someone else's schedule, pause. Ask yourself: Is this possible based on my schedule and ability to manage time? It may be better to inconvenience the person a little by saying you need an half hour more and be on time and reliable than be a half hour late and unreliable.

Put in a Margin

Another way to put yourself on a path to becoming a more reliable person is by building in extra time and planning for contingencies in case anything goes wrong.

> *ADHD dogged me but I fought the battle and won! The project I have been working on got done despite multiple computer meltdowns. When my computer ate my project, I still had my notes and a recent copy of the project printed out, just in case, so it was easy to reconstruct it.*

I had an inkling I might procrastinate on my project so I built in extra time and planned a backup, both of which really saved me. Worst case scenario I would have had an extra half a day to work on the project. The margin I created was a margin for error, just like a margin on a piece of notebook paper leaves you a space to write in. Yet I know that people affected with ADHD resist putting in a margin, which is why they are often late. Why the resistance to what could make life easier, less stressful?

Hating to Wait

People affected by ADHD tend to hate to wait, which is ironic because they make a lot of people wait on them due to their own lateness. If you see someone with ADHD who is not late and is waiting on someone or something they usually have an electronic device or another attention grabber like a book in hand. If they don't have anything with them, they look as though they have an internal itch they can't scratch.

Don't start anything new within 10 to 15 minutes of leaving your home. You are bound to get caught up in whatever activity you begin.

Since we hate to wait, we are often late. The lateness can happen in the morning or afternoon or evening. It most predictably happens whenever the ADHD-affected person is making their first exit from home for the day. No matter what time it is, there never seems to be enough time or the perfect time to leave, so they leave late.

Dealing with the Domino Effect

It is when they leave their home base late that a domino effect begins. People with ADHD tend to proceed as if they can still do everything they planned to do that day. For example, they may try to fit eight hours of appointments into seven hours. This just doesn't work. Granted, sometimes you can speed up, but usually not enough to get what you originally planned done. A 30-minute commute can't be done in 15 minutes (legally, that is) so something has to give.

Once you start the day late it is impossible to insert more time from somewhere else. If you started half an hour late, the domino effect is that you are a half hour late for everything throughout the day.

The best thing you can do once you realize you are behind is to decide what you are going to cut out of your day so that you can get back on schedule. As hard as it is, it's the only way to stop the domino effect.

An even better solution is to prevent this problem in the first place. To do this, give yourself a margin. Don't start anything new within 10 to 15 minutes of leaving your home because you are bound to get caught up in whatever activity you begin. Use those last few minutes to finish up or put away what you have been doing, and double check that you have everything you need for wherever you are going.

To ensure that you leave a margin, set your phone alarm to ring at both 15 minutes and at 5 minutes before the time you need to leave. The first alarm reminds you to finish up what you are doing or come to a good stopping place. The second alarm, at 5 minutes, means you *really must stop* and go immediately to the door.

Take a Break

Common wisdom is that if you want to get something done, keep working on it. Well, that is not the best way to get something done. Instead, if you want to get something done—take a break! Scientists have found this to be true.

Yes, that is right. Taking breaks is key to getting stuff done. Work for 30 to 50 minutes and then take a 15-minute break. After your break, get back to work. If you think this is hard to do, think of the alternative: keep working until you can't work any more on a project. Then the next day you are so burned out that you don't do any work on it—and that attitude can last for days. Instead, working with breaks means you will be able to sustain work on the project longer. Perhaps until the project is finished!

With some trial and error, you'll find whatever pace works best for you. No matter which approach you use, getting into the habit of taking breaks actually is hugely helpful for making you more productive and sustaining that productivity. (For apps that help you with taking breaks, see Appendix E.)

The Pomodoro Technique

Another way to do this is to use the Pomodoro technique. Pomodoro is especially helpful if you respond to visual stimuli. In this approach you work for 25 minutes and then take a 5-minute break.

On the Pomodoro website (www.pomodorotechnique.com) a clock tracks the time for you. Or you can order a Pomodoro clock to sit on your desk or wherever you are working.

Dealing with Activation

Those of us affected by ADHD can be a mass of contradictions: either wanting to nap all day like Winnie the Pooh once he has had his honey or being hyped up like Road Runner. When hyped, we feel like we can get anything done. When we are feeling soporific, the idea of accomplishing anything seems laughable at best.

How do you bestir yourself if you are in a Winnie the Pooh state and how do you calm yourself when you are in a Road Runner state? The solution to these problems often eludes me at the worst times.

Ironically, it's the activated Road Runner state that can lead to as many problems as when we're feeling like Winnie the Pooh.

The Night I Abandoned My Mother in a Train Station

I believe I am a good person and, most important, a good daughter. But I can remember that time when the good daughter label just didn't fit. Why? I left my mom overnight in a train station.

Whenever I tell this story to my clients, they say it makes them feel so much better. Never in all their lateness did they do something like this! While I am glad it makes them feel better, it felt pretty bad to me at the time.

I was living in Philadelphia at the time and my mother was taking the train up from Washington, D.C., to help me on weekends. This was a time in my life when I was physically disabled, so she came to help me grocery shop and run errands. It was truly generous of her to do this for me. I was thirty plus years old and she probably had thought she was done running errands for me a long time ago.

What happened that long ago Friday is that when I was about to leave to go to the train station to pick up my mom, the time pressure I felt did what it does for many people with ADHD—it stimulated me. Suddenly I felt that could finally get things done what I had been trying to do for days.

During that time my mother called me, repeatedly, and I kept saying I was about to leave. Each time I meant it sincerely. After hours of waiting it got late at night. She called and told me she was getting a cab to a hotel and she would see me in the morning. She was done for the day.

I knew I had blown it. I didn't understand why I hadn't just stopped and gone to the train station and picked her up. Now as an ADHD coach I understand. Having experienced so much failure, when you are finally feeling like you are getting things done, even if it is due to bad stimulation (being late), it is an addictive high. You are feeling success, an elusive experience for you. It is hard to stop.

It took much groveling and much time for me to overcome the guilt I felt for leaving my mother so long at the train station. I still wince when I think of it.

ADHD Brain Sequence

The brain sequence when I was planning to pick my mother up from the train station went something like this:

Got to hurry so I am not late => pressure => stimulation => activation

Result of activation => *I'll just do a quick pick up of my stuff before I leave* => *that was easy!*

Maybe I can get something else done? => feeling more pressure about time but also high from getting something done => *just one more thing, then I'll go* => *maybe one more* => rinse and repeat ad infinitum.

Being stimulated to act is great so long as it is at an appropriate time. Many of my coaching clients start getting to places on time once they commit to not starting anything new within 10 to 15 minutes of the time they need to leave home.

Using Hyperfocus to Your Advantage

I am under a crunch. Part of the reason is I am hoping to launch a new website and new programs this month, like on the 15th! It is now the 1st of the month. A lot of other people are involved in making this work but a large chunk is on me. I don't know if it is going to happen.

Feeling overwhelmed and stuck, unable to move forward, common with ADHD, has been haunting me. Well, not today! Today has been hyperfocus heaven! Sometimes when I have gone past the panic, past the worry, past the resistance, and past just about everything else, out of nowhere my hyperfocus zooms in and everything suddenly seems possible. I'm blasting away.

Hyperfocus can help you get a lot of things done, but this state of concentration does not last. It comes to an end, often before the work is done.

When we go into hyperfocus we can slam out work. But there is fear behind this—the fear that we won't be able to summon that hyperfocus when it's needed. We may be overwhelmed with work and don't feel that intense interest that helps us go into hyperfocus and work like nobody's business.

> ***Reflect on the progress you made and how making that progress made you feel: good, powerful, successful.***

How do you summon that hyperfocus when you need it? Here's what sometimes works for me. After I have had a day of slamming out work and I need another day like that due to deadlines or commitments, I sit back down where I worked the day before and think about how it felt getting all that work done. I reflect on the progress I made and how making that progress made me feel: good, powerful, and successful.

My body begins to feel that tingle of satisfaction again, a smile creeps onto my face and I think—I can kick some more butt today—just watch me! And, as if I were on a stage, I begin my grand performance of *This Is How You Slam Out More Work Today*.

I keep coming back to these reframes: feeling good, powerful and successful, performing, kicking butt, how it felt yesterday. Then all day I try to sustain my attitude as best I can, because your best is all you can do.

Whatever I do get done, I am grateful for. I do not think in terms of what was not done. Instead I prize the gift of what was done.

While this may not work exactly the same for you, if you have it in you to hyperfocus you can find a way to call on it when you need it.

Hyperfocus as a Curse

The ability to hyperfocus, seemingly a gift of ADHD, is also a curse. Hyperfocusing is becoming so focused on what you are doing that you lose track of time. I often hyperfocus when working on projects that interest me or reading books. I may get so involved in what I'm doing that I lose all track of time, read for 5 to 8 hours straight, and miss obligations I had during that time.

The ability to hyperfocus also makes people without ADHD doubt that there *is* such a thing as ADHD or doubt that you have it. Their argument is, well, you were able to stick to doing what you like to do, so you really shouldn't have a problem focusing on getting other things done. You are simply choosing not to or are lazy.

When someone affected by ADHD is working on something of intrinsic interest to them, their neurotransmitters process the correct chemicals efficiently. If what that person is working on is not of intrinsic interest, the chemicals dopamine and norepinephrine do not transfer efficiently between the neurotransmitters.

I think of it like train tracks. People without ADHD have train tracks that have been laid out to allow the trains to move efficiently. When there is a switch in the tracks used to re-route the trains, the re-routing works perfectly. For people affected by ADHD, their switching mechanisms are faulty and for that reason sometimes the trains don't run as smoothly. Sometimes the switching mechanism is so balky that goods fall out of the open top of the rail cars as they move along. Other times coupling and uncoupling the rail cars to move goods around to different destinations is not easy.

Don't Talk, Do—or, Not Having the Conversation with Yourself

Most people have heard about using positive self-talk to help us feel more valued. However, there are also conversations with ourselves that we shouldn't have.

Most of us resolve to do something to change. It may be a New Year's resolution or simply a stated intention. Whatever it is, we are trying to change something. Most often it is to start or stop habitual behavior. The question is, how do you change something that is deeply ingrained in you? There are no easy solutions. Change is hard to accomplish and difficult to sustain.

Block the internal dialogue and just do, do, do.

Each time I start to do something or not to do something, I have a conversation in my head:

> *Should I exercise now as I planned or maybe later when I feel more in the mood? But will I feel in the mood later? I really should do this now because this is when I said I would do it and I might not do it if I wait 'til later. But I really don't want to right now....*

And on it goes. The conversation has begun.

My simple suggestion is *do not engage in the conversation—at all.* Simply do the new action. Block the internal dialogue and just do, do, do. This is hard. It takes discipline. It also gets easier the more you do it. You have to keep your mind on the surface and not delve into the why's and what-fors. Just do what is on your schedule.

Once I start to exercise it becomes easier to continue. I will admit that sometimes I don't do my whole workout, but that is okay because I did some of it. And I did some of it at the time and place I scheduled to do it. Each time it gets easier.

If I don't do it, I don't berate myself. I let it go and either reschedule or wait for the next scheduled workout. I simply remind myself that this new routine is a work in progress and recommit myself. No negative self-talk. That kind of talk only gets in your way. It is another conversation not worth having.

Getting Mad to Help You Get Things Done

Things can get in your way and you can't get anything done. Things like phone calls, email notification pings, people you live with distracting you inadvertently, the general disorder of your environment, they all conspire against you! You have written on your calendar what you plan to do, but something gets in the way (maybe you!) and you don't get it done. You are frustrated and want to quit.

This may be the time you need to get your mad on. Getting mad, angry, and hostile can help you let out all of those frustrations. Again you'll say, *I will not be defeated,* while staying mad, feeding the anger, luxuriating in it. That is power you can use to look at your calendar again and focus on what needs to get done. As mentioned before, this works for only certain people. Also, as you start moving forward in what you want to get done, start transforming that angry energy into "I'm getting this done" energy and then into a celebratory energy.

Forget Perfect

Look at your calendar at least three times a day.

Your best is the best you can do.

To get more done, take breaks.

Set a timer to help you manage what you do.

Don't start anything new within 10 to 15 minutes of the time you need to leave home.

Chapter Four

Managing Your Relationship with Money

Yes, you do have a relationship with money. This chapter deals with it: budgeting, planning for the future, late payments, and setting up a system to manage and prevent the bad consequences that can result from ADHD symptoms. One disclaimer: I am not a money expert therefore anything regarding money written here is purely from a layman's point of view. Before doing anything regarding your financial situation check with a financial expert. The following information is not meant to be in lieu of expert opinion.

I grew up thinking men were bad with money and women were good with money. Imagine my surprise when I discovered that most people thought the exact reverse. In my family my mother managed the money because my father was not good at managing the family finances.

My father was more of a big picture kind of guy. In his work he made big financial decisions that affected many people. He took his responsibilities seriously and was excellent at making these decisions. But when it came to the family financial situation, he was out to lunch. Although he died in 1981 never diagnosed, my family and I believe it is likely he was affected by ADHD.

It is common for those of us affected by ADHD to be able to see the big picture but to fall apart when it comes to the details. I believe that is one of the reasons we have so many difficulties regarding money. Money is all about the details.

Budgeting

The first details to attend to include budgeting and tracking your expenses. Budgeting is a scary word for people affected by ADHD. We know we ought to be doing it. We might even like the concept of it, but following through on it stymies us. Budgeting is a system, and while systems intrigue us, we can make them awfully complicated and then either forget to use them or don't use them because of their complexity.

To get our financial house in shape we all need to have a budget—a simple budget—for three basic reasons:

- *We need to know for sure that more money is coming in than is going out.*
- *We need to be putting money away for the future so that we can maintain our lifestyle once we stop working.*
- *We need to create an emergency fund and grow it as our financial commitments grow.*

If technology helps you stay organized, use it. Many apps are available that can help you create and keep a budget (see the Appendix E for a list). The simpler the system the better and more likely you will use it.

Spending / Money Going Out

When developing a budget, create categories that break down how you spend money into groups so your money is easier to manage. Be careful not to start out with a million categories. The more categories, the greater the complexity. It's much better to stick to basics.

Below is an example:

- *Rent/Mortgage*
- *Insurance*
- *Medical*
- *Emergency fund*
- *Retirement fund*
- *Transportation*
- *Utilities*
- *Food*
- *Entertainment*
- *Clothing*
- *Miscellaneous*

A common mistake is to plan your monthly budget by taking your total annual expenses then dividing it by 12 to anticipate monthly expenses. However not all expenses are incurred in even monthly segments. Holiday and travel costs do not occur every month. You may have unexpected costs like repairing the dishwasher. Your car insurance may not be due monthly. These oversights can lead to unexpected expenses.

If you do not think it's realistic to expect that you will follow a budget or track expenses, I suggest using the envelope method. With this approach you use cash set aside by category as a way to manage your spending. You can find instructions easily by searching "money envelope system" online. There are also apps that mimic this approach. (See Appendix E)

Earning / Money Coming In

On the income side, record what you are taking in. If taxes are automatically taken out before you receive your paycheck, just record the amount of the check.

If you work for yourself or don't have taxes taken out, put aside money for estimated taxes. The best way to do this is to have your bank automatically deposit the appropriate amount into a savings account every time you deposit income. For example, if 15% of your income goes to taxes each year, have the bank deposit 15% of an income check into your savings account. This must be deposited in a savings account that you do not touch except for when you write your checks to the IRS and pay local taxes. If you pay your taxes on a quarterly schedule, you won't have that big tax bill due on April 15. Of course, please talk to a professional regarding any money issue, especially about your taxes.

Just as different expenses are due at different times and some months you'll have more expenses, income can vary as well. Some months bring in more money than others. For example, for salaried employees in some months there are two pay periods and in other months there are three pay periods.

Managing Credit Cards

What you spend using your credit card is part of your budget. The only difference is that payment is delayed until the end of the billing period.

Since interest on credit cards is incredibly high in most cases, do not spend more than you can pay off that month unless it is on an emergency expense. When you do not pay the entire amount due on your credit card each month, you are paying much more for whatever it is you think you bought at a great sale.

When you do not pay the entire amount due on your credit card each month, you are paying much more for whatever you think you bought at a great sale.

It is also important not to pay your credit card bills late because the interest charged on many credit cards increases once you have paid late. This means you are paying even more money for the convenience of using a credit card.

One approach to avoid the temptation of overspending or carrying credit card debt is to pay mostly by cash or check. The other is to just make sure to pay the balance off in full each month.

A good way to make sure you are really grasping how much you are paying in interest is to take your credit card statement (print it out if you don't receive it in the mail anymore) and highlight how much interest you paid that month. Keep doing it with each statement and start adding those amounts together. Getting a little scary isn't it?

Some people get radical and cut up all their credit cards. Don't do that. You may need one in case of an emergency. Do not, however, take on store credit cards because the interest is often even higher than regular credit cards.

If you have balances due on multiple credit cards see if you can switch all the balances to the credit card with the lowest interest rate to save yourself some money. Also if you have to pay off the debt on multiple credit cards, pay off the one with the highest interest first if you are unable to consolidate all the debt onto one low interest card.

Avoiding Late Payments

Avoid paying bills late. First off, late payments can begin to affect your credit rating and some credit cards increase interest after a late payment. For some of us, automatic withdrawal is a dream come true. For others of us, automatic withdrawal is a nightmare come true. For me, it is a nightmare because I lose track of how much I have in different accounts. Since I own my own business, I pay myself. Sometimes I forget to move the money to the correct account. Out of sight, out of mind for me. Getting a bill with a due date reminds me to deposit money from my business account to my personal account and then pay the bill. The lesson here is to know yourself and to do what works for you.

Impulsivity and Money

A component of ADHD is impulsivity. Impulse buying and spending plague many of us. With the advent of the Internet we don't even need to leave home to spend our money.

Do I really want to become someone who needs a new pair of shoes to feel better?

Ordering unplanned things off the Internet because we feel we need a treat or pick-me-up can turn into a dangerous, expensive habit. This is where it helps to be able to self-soothe without spending money. Get yourself out of a funk by talking or exercising rather than buying yourself out of it or by eating food when you are not hungry.

One of the ways I restrain myself from buying for comfort is to *question the act*. Do I really want to become someone who needs a new pair of shoes to feel better? Is there some other way I can get myself out of this mood or need to act impulsively?

Another thing I do is my own form of shock treatment. I figure out all the money that I still need to pay for the rest of the month. This includes any unpaid bills due that month, the cost of grocery trips, anticipated spending on special purchases or to get something fixed, the credit card balances, and any big money items coming up in the near future. I total the amount, making sure to overestimate each item's cost just in case.

Then I look up my bank checking account to see what the balance is. I subtract the total I came up for current and future expenses and take a pause. Is it really in my best interest to spend the money right now on the geegaw? Sometimes the answer is yes, but most often the answer at this point becomes no.

Saving Money

In 1990, at my first real job out of college, I was working for a non-profit and was paid $16,000 a year plus full insurance coverage. Despite the low salary, I managed to save money because my paycheck was directly deposited to my checking account except for $50 each pay period that was deposited into my savings account. The sum I had saved came in handy when I was laid off. It wasn't a lot, grant you, but any bit helps when you have lost your job.

One of the best ways to save money is to have a portion of your automatically deposited paycheck rerouted to your savings account. What you never have, you usually don't miss.

Contributing Towards Retirement

Years ago my mother was in line at a department store buying a wedding present for someone when she heard the woman in front of her talking to the clerk. The woman said how her son was a poor actor (financially poor!). Since I was a financially poor dancer my mom started to listen. The woman said instead of giving her son gifts he didn't need, she opened a Roth IRA account for her son and was putting a little into the account for each of his birthdays.

A Roth IRA has no tax implications for account holders until they retire and use the money. This meant his mother could put money towards his retirement—something he could not do owing to his financial situation—without his being burdened by an increased tax bill each year. Since he was unlikely to have much money upon his retirement, this not only helped him but also alleviated some of the mother's concern for his future.

My mother had similar worries so she opened a Roth IRA for me and put in the starting amount. Once something already exists it is easier to contribute to it.

Thinking that you need to put money away for your retirement and that you will just do it by adding more to your savings won't work for a couple of reasons:

- *The money will have virtually no growth so it is easy to think, why bother?*
- *If you do put money aside, you are likely to use those savings in an emergency or pseudo-emergency.*

It's better to open a Roth IRA because you are less likely to touch the money, it will not be taxed until you take the money out upon retirement, and it will help you differentiate between your emergency savings account and your retirement savings.

The later you start, the larger the amounts you will need to contribute. The goal is to increase the percentage in your retirement fund as you increase your income because your expectation of standard of living goes up as your income increases. It is much easier to adjust to a surplus of money in retirement than to adjust to a scarcity of money.

Creating an Emergency Fund

An emergency fund is supposed to cover six months of expenses according to the powers that be. This might not be a realistic goal for people affected by ADHD. I suggest you shoot for setting aside three months' worth of expenses in your emergency fund. This is thinking in an anticipatory way. This is important because as people affected by ADHD, we find that emergencies often happen to us and we're not prepared for them. Also, we are much more likely to lose our jobs than people who are not affected by ADHD. The emergency fund is therefore more likely to be necessary for us.

> *My car was 15 years old. I was happy that I didn't have to make monthly payments on it but at the same time I knew I needed to be thinking ahead—-putting aside money for the inevitable repairs and eventually for replacing the car with a new used car when the old one was no longer worth repairing.*

If you use some of that emergency money, start replacing it as soon as possible. Don't get complacent. There is no rule that says one emergency can't rapidly follow another. Also, as your income increases, make sure your emergency fund has contributions that reflect your new income.

Dealing with Finances When You Work for Yourself

People affected by ADHD are much more likely to become entrepreneurs than people not affected by ADHD. There are some particular considerations when setting up finances for a business. In addition to paying quarterly estimated taxes, you'll want to make sure that you have good financial records.

Separate Business and Personal Accounts

If you are self-employed, I encourage you to separate business financial accounts from personal accounts. I have a checking account for my business and one for my personal use, plus a savings account for each. Legally you don't have to have separate accounts, but come tax time it is much easier. I also find that writing a regular check from my business account to my personal account to pay myself helps me understand the real cost of doing business and the real cost of living. It also helps me avoid randomly taking money from my business when I need it. This is also good practice because you need to know at a certain point if your business can support you in a sustained fashion.

Facilitate Tracking with a Credit Card

If you are not good at keeping receipts, use a credit card for business expenses only. This will give you a good record of where your money went and will help you in doing your taxes when you have to categorize your expenses, if you do not already do that in your expense records.

Know Your Cash Flow

Look for patterns and observe what months require more money than other months. The most common mistake is to plan your monthly budget by taking your total annual expenses and income and then dividing by 12 to anticipate monthly expenses. That is not realistic when it comes to anticipating cash flow.

Some months cost more than other months and some months bring in more money than other months. For example, I have more income January/February and September/October than in July/August and November/December.

In terms of expenses, costs are rarely the same each month. Unexpected costs, like replacing office equipment will come up. Travel spending often varies by time of the year. Again, it's important to understand the patterns of your business and to think and plan ahead.

Hire Help; Spend Your Energy on Your Business

People affected by ADHD have trouble keeping up with the tedious tracking of expense reports, mileage, receivables, and the like. Don't let careless bookkeeping be the reason you don't succeed. If you have ADHD find someone to take care of the details so you can spend your time on revenue-generating activities and not be slowed down doing something you don't do well, probably do slowly, and waste a lot of time avoiding. It could make the difference in the success of your business. That person will also ensure regular billing, and bringing in receivables consistently allows for a constant cash flow that keeps your doors open and pays you without interruption.

Getting Your Taxes Done

You want to put it off and off and off. But that is not a good idea. So how do you get your taxes done or get your records prepared for someone else to get them done?

One approach is to get a shadow buddy. A shadow buddy is someone who keeps you company and helps you stay on task. It can be anyone; a friend, family member, another person affected by ADHD with whom you take turns being each other's shadow buddy.

The shadow buddy is there to encourage you and help you get back on task when you begin to wander. Your shadow buddy can remind you to take a break and then get back on task in a reasonable amount of time.

It helps if the shadow buddy understands people with ADHD and our avoidance issues. While I worked on preparing the tax information for my accountant, my shadow buddy read her book and glanced up occasionally to see if I was on task. She suggested a break when I was clearly beginning to run out of steam and then after about twenty minutes encouraged me to get back to work. She never told me what to do, which would have made me resistant, but instead asked questions like:

- *Where are you with recording your receipts?*
- *Do you feel you need a break or do you want to keep on going?*
- *Is there anything I can do to help?*
- *How long would you like your break to be?*
- *Is this a good time to get back to work?*

My shadow buddy left it up to me with no judgments about how I should be doing the work or using my time.

I try to reciprocate the help, either by being that person's shadow buddy, or by doing something else that is helpful to them. In this case, I helped my shadow buddy with her computer because that is where she has difficulty.

Taking Charge of Your Finances

Managing money is something that's hard for people with ADHD to do, whether it's because of difficulty with focusing on details, problems with setting up systems, lack of focus on the future, or impulsivity. But managing your money is critical to having the life you want now and in the future. There are ways to do it and to get help doing it even if you are affected by ADHD. Don't deny and don't delay!

Before all else, however, consult a financial advisor. I am providing knowledge based on my own experience and reading, but I am not an expert in this area. Your advisor is and can also give you advice that is specific to your situation.

Forget Perfect

Set up budgeting categories that work best for you, but make it simple so you'll actually use your budget.

Remember to set up an emergency fund.

Don't just learn to think about the future, act on it!

Set aside money for retirement.

Know your cash flow. It's not constant over time.

Find ways to soothe yourself without spending money.

Chapter Five

Setting Morning and Evening Routines

People with ADHD often have difficulty getting the sleep they need to be alert and focused. Some have trouble quieting down and getting to sleep in the evening at a reasonable hour. Others have trouble getting up and getting going in the morning, which can affect how prepared you are for the day ahead.

Lack of sleep makes ADHD symptoms much worse and can cause a downward spiral to the point where things seem hopeless. How can you prevent or reverse this spiral? Develop habits for the beginning and ending of the day. Just like brushing your teeth, getting to bed and then getting up and ready for the day are habits you can develop.

ADHD and Sleep Problems

I have always had trouble falling asleep and staying asleep, especially when I was little. My parents got tired of waiting up for me to fall asleep. They tried what they could to help me but nothing worked. Needing sleep themselves they decided to go to bed and check on me once in awhile throughout the night. Apparently I would wander the house at night and then fall asleep suddenly where I was at that particular moment. I discovered some pictures as an adult and they show me having fallen asleep so abruptly that I'm half on, half off couches and chairs like a discarded teddy bear.

Often we can't fall asleep and are resistant to going to bed. It can be very frustrating trying to quiet your mind enough at night to go to sleep. Some of us may need medication to sleep, which is tough to keep up with! Then, once we are asleep, we feel sluggish upon waking up.

Is It ADHD or Just Sleep Problems?

It has recently come to light that chronic sleep deprivation causes symptoms that mimic ADHD. Researchers are discovering that some people who were diagnosed with ADHD were simply suffering from chronic sleep deprivation and once properly treated, their ADHD symptoms receded.

Sleep is serious business for people affected by ADHD. Getting enough sleep every night can really help one manage their ADHD symptoms. It can be exhausting dealing with the effects of ADHD in our daily lives so it makes perfect sense that we need to devote extra time recharging ourselves through sleep or other renewing activities.

Getting to Sleep at Night

It is very common for people affected by ADHD to have trouble sleeping. As a coach, I work with many of my clients on what is called sleep hygiene. Sleep hygiene is preparing for and getting the best sleep you can get.

Part of getting a good night's sleep is managing what you do prior to going to bed and setting up routines that help you get a good night's sleep. First, you'll want to pick a time to begin your ending process for the day. This may include a 5- to 7-minute walk-through of your home, picking up things that are in the wrong rooms and moving them to the correct rooms. Follow this with deciding what you will be wearing the next day and laying out everything you will need on a chair to be ready for you in the morning. If you have a bag or briefcase to take to work in the morning, have it packed and ready by the door. What is happening is that with these actions you are presetting for the morning, when you are less likely to remember things or be as alert about what is going on as you are in the evening.

Don't Let Yourself Get a Second Wind

Many people affected by ADHD are night owls, or so they claim. I think some truly are but others simply are not allowing themselves to quiet down as they prepare for bed. They then stay up long enough to reach their second wind, making it harder to go to sleep. If you go to bed before your second wind you will not run into that extra burst of energy that can keep you awake.

Contributing to keeping you awake at night may be a whole host of things: using electronic devices, having phone conversations, exercising, or having sugar or caffeine late in the day.

When you stay on the computer, tablet, cell phone, or other electronic device right up to the very last minute you go to bed, or even while you're in bed, the light from the digital screen keeps you awake rather then settling you down.

If you talk on the phone late at night, when you're having conversations, you can get excited and your mind starts thinking about many different things. You have reengaged yourself rather than quieted yourself down.

Exercising actually increases your energy rather than tiring you out. It is also not good to eat sugary snacks right before bedtime because sugar also gives you a punch of energy. Finally, do not drink anything that has caffeine in it after 4 p.m. or 5 p.m. depending on when you go to sleep.

Here are some other ways to help you get a good night's sleep:

- *Decide what time (a reasonable time!) you want to turn out your lights.*
- *Take a moment to check your schedule for the next day.*
- *Make your 3- to 5-item to do list for the next day.*
- *Make sure you're in bed at least 30 to 45 minutes before lights out.*
- *If you have been prescribed medication to help you sleep, take it 20 to 30 minutes before lights out.*
- *Do not take your electronics with you to bed. Light from the screen will keep you awake (there are screen covers you can get that diminish the type of light the screen emits that keeps you awake).*
- *Listen to music, read (print book, magazine, newspaper) or similar activity.*
- *Have a pen and sticky notes by your bed for any ideas that come to you during the night (this way you will not have to try and remember for the morning or get up and risk waking yourself up further).*
- *Turn your lights out at the designated time.*
- *If need be, have ambient music on to help you sleep.*

If you wake up in the middle of the night do not start on the computer or other digital equipment. It will wake you up rather then lull you back to sleep.

Getting Going in the Morning

Getting up and going in the morning can be difficult for people affected by ADHD. Many of my clients have come to me having lost their jobs because they simply were not able to regularly get to work on time. There are ways to set yourself up for getting into your day without delay.

As discussed in the last section, a successful beginning of the day begins the night before. By going to bed at a reasonable time and doing it properly, you have a better chance of falling asleep easily and having good rest by the time morning comes. In addition, with everything for the morning prepped—your outfit for the day laid out, your bag packed and by the door, a lunch to take out of the refrigerator—you don't have so much to look after in the morning.

Breaking the Night Owl Habit

If you are in the habit of going to bed really late and want to break that habit, start slowly and begin to move your bedtime about 15 minutes earlier every few days or every week. Keep your bedtime and wake-up time consistent, whether it is a weekday or weekend. If your bedtimes vary greatly it will make it much harder on you to set a regular sleep time and be able to actually go to sleep then.

If you have debilitating sleep issues, talk to your doctor (your GP) about whether it would be worth it to have a sleep study done. They are expensive and generally need to be prescribed by your doctor to be covered by insurance. Even without a sleep study, a sleep specialist may be able to make suggestions that may help you.

You looked at your calendar and made a short to do list before you went to sleep so you know what the day will bring as much as possible. Doing this means that any adjustments you need to make in the morning can be done quickly.

Get into a Routine

Everyone has a particular order of how they like to do things in the morning. Here are some things that I consider must-do's (and must don'ts!).

Taking Your Meds

If you are supposed to take medication for your ADHD in the morning and you have trouble waking up and getting started here is a tip: Set two alarms—one for when you need to get up and one for a half hour earlier than that. Put your ADHD med(s) and some water at your bedside in the evening. When the first alarm goes off in the morning, take your med(s) and let yourself go back to sleep until the second alarm wakes you up to get up. Many people find that taking their pill(s) before they get out of bed makes getting out of bed easier because their medicine is already working.

Activate Yourself

If you are still dragging, find another way to activate yourself. For example, take your shower next.

> *I am feeling really sluggish after I have finished washing my hair (the last thing I do in the shower) so I step from under the shower head and turn the hot water down some and then stick my head back under the water as though I am rinsing my hair again. The cool water on my head for a few seconds gets me moving without having to put my whole body under. I suffer but not completely because it is only my scalp that gets the hit of cool water. Sometimes you got to do what you got to do!*

Eat Breakfast

It's important to eat breakfast because it provides energy. Include in your breakfast some protein because it helps people with ADHD function better—and be sure to go easy on the sugar.

Leave Neatly

As you go through your morning routine, try not to leave in your wake a trail of destruction, including in the kitchen. This is because (a) you won't clean up after yourself when you get home, and (b) it's no fun getting home in the evening facing more chaos.

Be Careful about Checking Email

If you must check your email in the morning get out of bed first, because if you do it while in bed you may not get out of your bed for a while and will lose momentum. I believe you should wait until you are dressed so if time gets away from you it is not a total catastrophe. Since you are already dressed you can dash out the door if need be.

Stay Focused on Getting Out the Door

Critical to getting out of the door on time is staying focused on this one task—getting out the door on time. To be successful, do not start roaming the Internet or playing computer games. Just about every client I have had who got in trouble for being late to work played computer games or roamed the Internet before they left for work. The thinking is, *I will just play one game while I am eating breakfast or before I get out of bed.* There is no such thing as playing one game or spending only 5 minutes on the Internet for someone affected by ADHD. It is just not possible for most of us. Why put yourself in a situation where you are likely to succumb and lose track of time?

Another thing to watch out for as you are leaving is starting to do things you have been meaning to do around your home. For those of us with ADHD, when we are starting to be a little late and feel the pressure of lateness, that pressure stimulates us. When we are stimulated we activate and are able to do things. (That is how stimulants work for people affected by ADHD. They stimulate us, making us able to accomplish things.)

We see things we think we can do in just a minute or two. In reality it is going to take longer, but we don't think about that. We stop and do it. I am then thinking *That that was really successful. I got it done quickly. I will do something else, and it will only take a minute more...*and so it goes. An hour later you realize you are going to be in big trouble if you go to work at this point since you are so late. Your solution is to call in sick, which is also going to get you in trouble because you have already used up your sick days because of the days like this happening to you. Furthermore, you are losing credibility at your job so your boss is not going to be inclined to help you out.

Sample Morning Plan

First alarm: take meds

Second alarm: get out of bed

Put coffee on

Eat breakfast while reviewing that day's planning calendar

Shower

Dress

Make sure you have everything you need for the day by the door

If time, quick pick up

Leave

Mornings are a danger zone for us. Make a plan, write it down, and follow it. Try it for awhile. If it works, keep at it. If not, make adjustments until you have a routine that works for you, then stick to that. Also figure out what things you can drop from your routine if you are running late. This way if you are running late you don't have to think about what to do. You have already made that decision. All you need to do is follow what you have decided in advance.

Forget Perfect

Turn off all screens at least 40 minutes before going to bed.

Get ready for your day the night before—set out clothes, etc.

Follow a plan for going to bed and getting up.

Don't overactivate before you leave your home in the morning. You will start to do things, get distracted, and leave late.

Good sleep hygiene. Treat it just like you do brushing your teeth.

Chapter Six

Simplifying Daily Life

For those of us with ADHD, a rule of thumb is simpler is better. If we can make daily life simpler and easier by developing schedules to take care of routine tasks, we are already succeeding at this. Doing so will give us more time to build the life we want. This chapter gives approaches, ideas and techniques for simplifying your daily life—and avoiding needlessly complicated systems that we can't sustain.

Taking Meds

If you are on medication, make a schedule and follow it so that you take your medications at the right times each day. Keep it simple. Carry a pill case containing your meds, and set your phone alarm. If you do forget to take your meds and take a stimulant late in the day, it may keep you up at night. Check with your doctor about what to do if you miss a dose.

Also, set up a schedule for filling and picking up your prescription. Set a reminder on your calendar for ordering your prescription each month and for going to the pharmacy to pick up your meds. Be sure to give yourself a couple of days' leeway in case things don't run like clockwork. Put any meds that qualify for automatic refill on automatic refill. Don't wait until the last minute because your pharmacy may be out of your medication. If you do wait until the last minute, have the contact information for a fallback pharmacy, one that your primary pharmacy can contact if they are out of your meds.

You may be taking your meds during the week to be more effective at work but when you're home on the weekends you may feel more "you" without the meds. Is this really fair? Shouldn't your family also get the benefit of your attentiveness and ability to get things done? This is something to discuss with your family. It affects them, not just you.

Why a Keeping to a Schedule for Meds Is Important
Each ADHD medication has a certain length of efficacy, and because our bodies are all different, lengths of efficacy may be different for different people. Find out the length of time for each medicine that has been prescribed for you. If it is 10 hours, then be mindful of which 10 hours of the day you need the benefit of that medicine.

If you are on a short-acting medicine and need to take it several times a day, set an alarm on your phone to remind you to take your med at the right times. Others might take a long acting med and then a short acting med in the late afternoon. Again, set your alarm. Be smart - keep in mind that stimulants keep people awake. If you forget to take your short-acting med in the afternoon – don't take it at 5 p.m. or later because it will interfere with your getting to sleep.

Clearing Out Clutter

The world shifted, and I fell this morning. I fell on Monday too. I am getting suspicious. Maybe the world isn't shifting, and I am falling because there is so much stuff on my floor. The books, papers, bags, notebooks, and newspapers on my floor may be why I keep slipping.

I did what any adult would do after these two incidents. I called my mommy! Her response was to ask me why I didn't pick up the stuff after my first fall on Monday. She obviously doesn't have ADHD. I hate logical answers! Although my back was aching and my arm hurt I cleared my floor.

One of the biggest challenges for people with ADHD is managing the clutter that surrounds them. When you walk into a cluttered room, it becomes a distraction and adds clutter to your mind. The underlying message is "you should be taking care of this." As a result, clutter makes it harder for you to focus on the task at hand and adds stress that you might not be aware of. You are living with this nagging feeling that you should be taking care of this. So how *do* you take care of clutter?

A first step in dealing with clutter is to become a tyrant. You don't want to be a tyrant to your family or friends, but a tyrant about what comes into and what goes out of your home. I use the word tyrant because that is what you must be to help yourself and the people you live with. Clutter cannot be solved if there are more things than a space can hold—and you can't clean until you remove the clutter from the space to be cleaned.

You must banish from your kingdom anything that doesn't fit or have its own home.

Every item in your home needs to have its own home, a place where the item lives when not in use. Once all those places in your home are taken, any stuff left over has to go. If you have more stuff than you have places to store it, you have a problem. This is where being a tyrant comes in handy. You must banish from your kingdom anything that doesn't fit or have its own home. If something comes into your kingdom, the tyrant in you either needs to throw it out of the kingdom or throw out something else to make room for the new item in the kingdom.

You remove things from your kingdom by giving them away to friends, neighbors, or charity, or by putting into the trash items that are no longer usable. When storing items, do not stack them unless you are stacking the same item. Otherwise you will have to pull the item from the middle or bottom of the stack and the stack will probably fall over. In addition it is difficult to put the item back because you will have to lift the stack up to insert the item into its proper place, which is something you are not likely to do.

We tend not to put back the things we get out. You get something out because you want to use it but when you are done with the item there isn't a lot of incentive to put it away, especially if it's in a hard-to-get-to spot.

Many clients have found *www.FlyLady.net* a helpful site. Here you can find support and suggestions on how to keep your home clean. Other clients have found it a bit overwhelming because of the level of detail. See Appendixes C and E for books and apps to get help with this.

If you have to chose always make something easier to put away than it was to get out. When you need something, you will go through the effort to get it. Putting things away lacks the desire component of needing something. Therefore, the easier it is to put away, the greater the possibility that it will in fact get put away.

Getting Rid of Paper

If sleep is the bane of existence for people affected by ADHD, the second runner up would be paper.

I went to three conferences in three weeks, each conference was filled with sponsors handing out materials left and right. What do I do? I take it all. Then I get home and can't throw it out. What if I need that information in the future, like twenty-five years from now? What if the Internet goes down and the brochure is the only way I will ever find that book cover for when I write my great American novel? ... It could happen ... some day!

I actually have no interest in writing a novel but things change, right? Anyway, that is how the thinking goes for many people affected by ADHD when trying to throw out paper. *I might need it in the future!*

This is a phrase that becomes a not-so-helpful mantra for people like us. You need to challenge this statement by asking yourself could I find the information another way in the future? Would this information even be current in the future or is it time sensitive?

One thing is for sure: the more you toss, the easier it is to toss more. If you can get yourself in the flow of tossing things you will find it easier to let go of more things, paper and otherwise.

Finding Files Quickly by Creating Simple Systems

Often due to our ADHD, it is difficult to quickly put our hands on papers and files when we need them. We don't know where things are because we don't put them away where they belong after we use them. The first step is to make things easy to put away in assigned easy-to-spot homes. If you are going to put something in a container make it a clear container or clearly label it. Make the label large enough to be read from a few steps away.

If you need paper files as I do for my handwritten notes that go in my client files, use an open file system. I don't recommend filing cabinets for people with ADHD. It becomes a wasteland just taking up space. I use steel-based frames that have a divider every couple inches so that my files all stand up on open shelves (wire organizer from MMF Industries). Each file folder is the kind you see in most doctors' offices, with the tab on the end not the side. They're called *end tab* folders. This makes each file easy to read from the bookshelf.

Don't worry about making pretty labels for your files; worry about function first. Dwelling on making your files look stylish will just slow you down or get in the way of you getting the task done. Simply write labels on the file tabs in big letters. Don't get caught up in pretty, get caught up in done!

If you don't put something away after you use it, add a 5- to 10-minute end-of-the-day pick-up to your routine, or at least get items in the general vicinity of where they live. This won't completely solve the problem but at least it increases the chances of quickly putting your hands on what you are looking for.

Using a Shadow Buddy to Help Clear Clutter

I have a goal for Monday. It's to clear away all the random paper on my desk, hutch, trunk, printer, and copy machine. I am going to do this with the help of a shadow buddy.

My shadow buddy will help me retake my room. I will admit it is embarrassing that I still need her to come every once and a while to help me retake the same area, but this is my pattern. When working, I just put papers aside when I am done with them. Then they breed. Not my fault.

My shadow buddy is good at getting me to throw out unnecessary paperwork that I seem to cling to and to actually make files and not just stack up all the papers.

I realize I should be trying to go paper free, all digital, but I am too old for that, set in my ways, all forty plus years of them. But I am trying.

Creating a Home for Each Thing

Making homes for items helps you put them away and know where to find them. While this sounds obvious, it can take time to think through and try different places until you find the right place for the right item. You want to have homes for everything in your house, but most importantly you want to have homes for things that you take in and out of your house.

Launching Pads

In the ADHD world, a launching pad refers to a place that is designated to hold what you need when you leave your home. Just like an astronaut on a launch pad goes through a checklist to make sure everything is ready to go, your launch pad is where you put everything you need before you go. Where your launch pad is located and what it holds will vary from person to person but usually it is right by the front door or the kitchen door or wherever you exit and enter your home.

The number one thing the launch pad holds is your keys. Keys deserve a special home. Without keys you can't get into your home or start your car (if you have one). Therefore it is important that your keys have a home in your home and in a bag or pocket when you are out and about. It is also important that someone you trust has a copy of your home key and car key in case of emergency. For some people the launching pad might also hold their mobile phone and wallet.

When you are at home the things that belong on the launch pad stay on the launch pad. If they are needed elsewhere, then put them back on the launch pad immediately after you are done with them. If I need a credit card while I am home, I go to the launching pad I have for my bag, get the card, use it, and them immediately return it to my bag on its launch pad.

If you carry a bag or a purse you might not want that to be the first thing people see upon entering your home. In that case create a secondary launching pad in a place that you always go by when you leave your home.

Upon entering my home, directly across from the front door is a small set of drawers and on top of it is a little heart-shaped dish my nephew made when he was younger. That is the launching pad for my keys. Every time I go out I know my keys are there. When I come in my keys go there without fail. If I am carrying groceries I may walk to the kitchen and dump my groceries, but then I immediately put my keys on the launching pad before I do anything else.

Make strict use of the launching pad as a rule you promise not to break. It will take some practice but once you get it down, those awful moments of forgetting your keys, your wallet, or some other important thing are relegated to the past.

One final note: if you need to remember to take something special with you the next time you leave, just put it next to your launch pad. Library books placed next to your keys are more likely to go out the door with you than if you leave the books in your living room.

Homes for Action Items

It is also important to create homes for items that require action. For example, I put clothes that need dry cleaning in a place clearly visible to me when I am leaving my bedroom. With just a glance I know if it is time to drop off my dry cleaning. Either I have accumulated enough to make the trip worthwhile, or there is something in the pile I will need soon. By placing them in a special place, I know when I have to act.

Cleaning

The best way I know how to clean is to keep each activity short and contained. This means do not schedule three hours to clean once a week. Instead, plan to clean in short spurts. Break down the areas of your home to be cleaned, or break down the types of tasks such as mopping, vacuuming, laundry, dusting, etc.

Use a timer and set it for 15 to 20 minutes. Work furiously while the timer ticks away. Once the alarm rings, stop. It is much easier to contemplate doing 15 minutes of cleaning than hours or a whole day's worth. Starting is easier when the end is in sight.

Laundry

Always have a place and a container for your dirty laundry. If you fling your clothes off and leave them on the floor, then you don't know what is clean and what is dirty. If you think it is too much effort to put your dirty laundry in one place, I would ask: isn't it more work to wash it all because you are not sure what is clean and what is dirty?

I also suggest an intermediary clothing site. This intermediary site is for clothes that you have worn once and can wear again before they need to be cleaned. Knowing I am unlikely to put the clothes away, I have found an intermediary site helpful in keeping clothes off the floor and the furniture in my bedroom. Of course, put away clean clothes immediately after the laundry is done or it won't happen.

Farming Out Regular Tasks

If you can afford it, farm out as many things as you can. Here are a few ideas:

- *Take your laundry to a Laundromat that will do your laundry charging you per pound.*
- *Hire someone to come in and clean. If you can't afford to have them come every week, what about every other week? You do light pick up and cleaning throughout the month; they do the rest. But if you are going to do that make sure you have enough underwear to last for two weeks if the person is also going to do your laundry!*

Setting Up Repeats

An important habit that can simplify your life is setting up a plan for accomplishing recurring tasks or activities. This is what I call your repeats, activities that are repeated, typically weekly or monthly.

Weekly and Monthly Repeats

Weekly repeats could include grocery shopping, vacuuming, or taking out the garbage. Monthly repeats could be picking up your prescription refills at the pharmacy, taking clothes to the dry cleaner, or dropping accumulated stuff off at a charity. These reoccurring activities should be pre-scheduled and land at the same time each week or month.

Every Friday my mother and I go grocery shopping. It is a great arrangement. Taking her forces me to buy my groceries on a regular schedule so that I don't go impulse shopping when I am starving and end up with just cupcakes and peanut butter in the kitchen cabinets. Since I know I am going shopping every Friday, I know how much food to buy. This results in less wasted and spoiled food and better eating habits. It also gives us a regular time to visit with each other.

Making Repeats Work

Repeats only work if you schedule them consistently and make doing them a habit. Sometimes you will fail, but that isn't a reason to give up. Just start again after you evaluate possible reasons for failure. Is the day you are choosing to do something a poor choice? Are you unrealistic about the time you need to do the repeat? Are you planning to do the repeat after you have done another repeat that historically tires you out so that it is unlikely you will have the energy to mow the lawn next?

When my mother and I first started our Friday morning forays, I regularly set up phone meetings at 1pm or 2pm but I would either miss the call or forget about the call. I learned if I was going to take my mom grocery shopping and run other errands at 10:45am, then come home and unpack my groceries, I was unlikely to make or remember the calls. So, I shifted what I scheduled on Fridays. Before 10:30am I could do calls and then I schedule non-time-sensitive activities like paperwork for the early afternoon.

Creating Visible Reminders for Your Repeats

Be sure to create charts for your weekly and monthly repeats. This will help make what you need to do on a regular basis visible. Post your charts in an accessible place, where you will see them regularly. This is especially helpful when you are entering things in your calendar or checking your calendar for what is coming up.

I make my charts in Excel on my computer, but you can make a chart with just a piece of paper and ruler. (Write in pencil at first until you have a routine that works.) The charts below are samples. Create what works for you.

Weekly Repeats

Mon	Tues	Wed	Thurs	Fri	Sat	Sun
Paper-work Exercise	Clean Bath-room	Exercise	Volunteer (1/2 day)	Grocery Shopping Exercise	Clean Living Room	De-cluttering

Monthly Repeats

	Mon	Tues	Wed	Thurs	Fri	Sat	Sun
Week 1				Dry Cleaning			
Week 2						Pay Bills	
Week 3				Dry Cleaning			
Week 4						Pay Bills	

Quarterly Repeats

Spring	Spring cleaning, planting garden, wardrobe changeover
Summer	School preparation, scheduling extra-curricular activities
Fall	Holiday preparation, wardrobe changeover, winterizing
Winter	Planning Summer vacation, put up and take down holiday decor

Planning Meals and Shopping for Groceries

Getting organized in the kitchen is often the first step to creating a cycle of grocery shopping, making healthy meals that can be pulled together quickly, and saving money.

Eating Out Costs Money

One incentive for preparing meals at home is that you can save money. If you wonder where your money goes, check out how much money you are spending eating out or ordering in food. It may be more than you think. Those of us with ADHD rarely plan ahead enough to start preparing our food before we are hungry. This results in not wanting to eat anything that requires prep time. We want to eat now and we may not feel like putting forth the effort that is required to make a meal.

That is why it is important to choose easy meals that require very little prep time and need only a few simple ingredients that are easy to put together. The simpler you keep things, the greater likelihood they will get done. If you make more than you will eat, you can put the extra in portion-sized microwavable containers. This will give you some quick and easy meals for lunch or dinner with little effort.

Setting Up Your Kitchen

In setting up your kitchen, put everything as close as possible to where you will use it. Store pots and pans near your stovetop and oven. Store glasses near the refrigerator because most likely what you drink comes out of the refrigerator. Mugs go near the coffee pot and microwave-safe dishes near the microwave. Sometimes your kitchen design will prevent you from putting things in a convenient place. In that case, just do the best you can.

A mantra for this chapter is *the easier something is to put away, the more likely it will be put away*. Try to avoid stacking items on top of each other unless they are the same item. For example, if you have to choose between the effort of getting something out versus putting that thing away, always make something easier to put away than it is to get out. This is true for everything in your home, not just what is stored in the kitchen.

Planning Healthy Meals

People affected by ADHD may be more likely to be obese. It is still early in the research, but some experts attribute this tendency to poor eating habits and failing to exercise. I believe the reason for this is that those of us diagnosed with ADHD are more likely to eat processed food because it is hard for us to plan ahead.

If we don't plan ahead, we won't have the ingredients we need to make healthy meals. Even if we do have the right ingredients on hand to make something nutritious, we tend to go for something that involves no work or waiting time. Planning ahead and following through are just not our forte. For those of us who do manage to plan ahead, we often make the process needlessly complicated, have unrealistic goals, or follow someone else's plan that is not right for us. For example, many people go wrong when they plan meals because they create a menu of things they don't normally eat. Then the food goes to waste.

My suggestion is to become an investigator! For two to four weeks keep a food diary and write down everything you eat during each day. Look at the list of foods you have eaten and then pick the meals that are the easiest to make, that you like to eat, and that are healthy for you. If you don't end up with many meals, look at what you ate the last few weeks that was not good for you or easy to make. Think about what could be a satisfying substitute that also meets the criteria of easy to make, something that you like, and that is healthy.

Next, get some index cards and write down one meal per card along with all of its ingredients (for apps that do this, see the Appendix E). Each week, select the meals for the week from the pile of index cards. Do not try more than one new meal a week. Take those cards to the market so you buy the ingredients you need. Gradually increase your number of meal cards for greater variety. Remember you don't need complicated recipes.

Grocery Shopping

Plan your trip to the grocery store. Try to go shopping just once a week—and always have a list! Going to the grocery store without a shopping list, even if it is just a mental one, is dangerous. Why? Because you are likely to:

- *spend too much money*
- *get a lot of crappy food*
- *end up with either not enough food for the week and/or too much food, which means much of it will go bad in your refrigerator*

Plan your meals for the week (see Planning Healthy Meals). Make a list of the foods you will need for the meals or take the recipe cards with you. Remember to check the ingredients you already have so you don't double buy. Be sure to add some healthy snack foods. We are people of impulse, and that includes eating.

To save you from having to run more errands, add to your list any other things you need that you can get at the grocery store, like papertowels or toothpaste. Before I go grocery shopping, I do a quick run through my home, checking on my stock just as a store might do. I look to see if I have at least enough for the week.

Basic Shopping List (Sample)

Groceries • Paper towels • Toilet paper • Cleaning supplies for the home • Birthday or holiday cards (I have been saved a time or two by my grocery store) • Toiletries • School or office supplies • Light bulbs • Flowers • Cosmetics • Health supplies

Be careful not to overstock on some things. It wastes space, contributes to clutter, eliminates cash on hand, and we may never use the extra stock. A bargain isn't a bargain if you wouldn't have bought it anyway.

To help sustain your effort to systematize your grocery routine, do your grocery shopping on the same day each week. Make it one of your weekly repeats. Even better, get together with a buddy and shop together on the same day. Having a weekly appointment with someone to do your grocery shopping will help you stick to your plan. If for some reason the day you plan to shop does not work for you or your buddy, schedule an alternative time as soon as you know the regular time won't work. You want to make sure that it still happens that week.

If you do drop the routine, simply pick up where you were as soon as possible. Don't waste time judging yourself. Get back on track instead.

Setting Up Habits and Systems

As mentioned under Setting Up Your Kitchen, if there's a theme in this chapter, it's that you simplify by setting priorities, developing habits, and setting up and following systems.

Hook a New Habit to One You Already Have

The easiest way to develop a habit is to hook a new habit to one you already have. Some of my clients, before they go to bed, place their medicine and a glass of water by their bed so the first thing they do upon getting up is take their medicine. This is especially helpful to those of us who wake up extremely groggy in the morning. Set an alarm, wake up, take your pills, and then go back to sleep for 20 or 30 minutes until your second alarm goes off. It will be easier to get up then because your ADHD medication will already be working.

Another example of hooking one habit to another is that my mother may add to our weekly trip to the grocery store a visit to the dry cleaners, bank, pharmacy or library when needed. All I have to do is tell her what else I need to do when I think of it. Her knowing I need to go somewhere in addition to the grocery store makes it more likely that it will happen, particularly because when things are spoken aloud to others, it increases the likelihood they will get done.

Ditching Needlessly Complicated Systems

When creating systems, those of us with ADHD tend to make them needlessly complicated. While we think a more complicated system is better, the exact opposite is true: the more complicated it is, the less likely we are to use it.

When I used to pay all my bills by check, I kept a folder for each vendor: phone company, gas company, each credit card company, landlord/rental company, car insurance, health insurance, etc. However, my mother kept telling me to have one folder per year and just put each bill I paid on top of the previous bill I had paid because it was more likely I would get the bills filed and they would be easy to find.

I resisted for a long time but finally tried her system. The true test was when I had to find an old phone bill. I thought *Ha! Now, I will prove that her system stinks. It will take me forever to find this old bill.* It took me less than a minute. The bills were in a basic chronological order so all I had to do was go back in time.

Even now with paying the bills electronically I use my mother's method. My paid bills and business receipts get filed, reducing the chaos on my desk. They get filed because it takes the same amount of time to toss the bill on my desk as it does to toss it in the folder.

Each year I have a great reference for my taxes if I have a question that my spreadsheets can't answer. A copy of each year's tax returns and related spreadsheets go on top on the year's paid bills, and the file is put away until I am legally allowed to shred all but the tax returns.

The point here is KISS – keep it simple sweetheart. Not only did the simplified system fix the problem that the complicated system was not achieving, it also led to solving another issue in a simple way: keeping my annual taxes and supporting documents organized and together.

Getting Routine Tasks Done

On big, important things I usually don't have much difficulty getting started. It is the tedious day-to-day stuff that can be hard for me to get done on a regular basis. That means things like paying bills, filing, getting packages mailed, responding to a request that I am not really excited about, and opening mail in a timely fashion.

I find that this is true for a lot of people with ADHD. To people without ADHD, it seems that these things are simple and we should just do them. But it is not that easy. If it were easy for us we wouldn't have ADHD!

To deal with these tasks I suggest two approaches:

1. Set aside a day each week (say, Monday) for tasks you tend to put off (for me, it's paperwork).
2. Try to deal with things you come in contact with in the moment rather then setting them aside for later. If I get a file out, I try to put it away when I am done with it rather than just adding it to the stack beside my desk.

A key to making this all happen is having a schedule and a home for everything. If you're not sure where something belongs, you won't bother to put it away.

Use a Shadow Buddy

Having a partner often helps people get things done. This is especially true if you have ADHD. Often called a shadow buddy this is a person who stays with someone with ADHD who is trying to accomplish a task they have been having a hard time either getting started, finishing, or both.

Directions for the Shadow Buddy

If you are using a shadow buddy let them know what you need from them. The shadow buddy is usually a non-ADHD person, and this is what they need to know:

Be present. Don't do anything other than help keep the ADHD person on task in a gentle nonjudgmental, supportive way.

You may have to help the ADHD-affected person figure out where to start. You won't necessary directly tell the ADHD-affected person what to do because people all do things differently and different minds have different processes. Instead, ask the ADHD-affected person questions to help them hone in on what they are trying to achieve and what their ideas are for how to go about it. You might list a few options and allow the ADHD-affected person either to choose one or come up with their own approach. Don't get caught up with what is the most efficient way. Someone affected by ADHD has the right to do something any way he or she feels comfortable doing it.

Getting Regular Exercise

Another great buddy to have is an exercise buddy. Science has proven that exercise releases chemicals into the brain in the same way stimulants do for people affected by ADHD. Regular exercise is important and is one of what I call the "Five Fingers" of ADHD treatment (for more on the five fingers, see Appendix A).

Regular exercise is hard for most people and then add on top of that the difficulty people affected by ADHD have with doing things consistently. That said, having an exercise buddy can make a real difference in whether you actually show up to do a workout, play a sport, or do any other activity that gets your heart rate up for a period of time. Of course if you have not exercised recently, find out from your doctor if there is any reason you shouldn't be exercising or if there are certain types of exercise that would not be good for you.

> *I had always thought that after I retired from my first career as a dancer, I would bike ride for fitness. Oddly enough, without prompting my doctor said not to ride regular bikes after my back surgery and if I wanted to ride a bike it had to be a recumbent one. Check with your doctor before starting to exercise, and tell them what kind of exercise you are thinking of doing.*

Tips for Getting It Together

I am an ADHD coach and, yes, I can get overwhelmed. When that happens, I remind myself to make a list, prioritize, and look for things I can drop or save for later. Then I approach each thing one at a time and do the best I can do in the time I have allotted for it. I don't get stuck using all my time on one thing and leaving other important things undone. Sometimes good enough is the best you can do, and it frees you to accomplish more. Another thing I do is remind myself of things that help me get it together. Here's one of those lists:

- Make a home for everything. That means a huge de-cluttering first!
- Use a shadow buddy when needed. Their presence keeps you on task to get it done. Family and friends are good shadow buddies.
- Make simple task lists. These lists keep you focused on what needs to get done.
- Have lists and schedule repeat activities that you have trouble remembering. For example, have a permanent packing list for travel that includes everything but clothes. This includes things like cell phone charger, contact lens solution, etc.
- Hire or trade out things you can't or won't do. You might hire someone twice a month for an hour to do your bills and filing, someone to clean once a week or every other week.
- Use an organizer or planning calendar ruthlessly! Paper, computer, or cell phone—keep it with you and check it multiple times a day. Write everything in it. Look ahead a week and a month so you know what is coming down the road so there are no surprises (for more on organizers and planning calendars, see Chapter 5).

Plan and Prioritize Your Tasks by Your Energy

Those of us with ADHD tend to become more easily distracted the later in the day it is. For that reason, plan the tasks that require the most energy when you have the energy to do them. And if you find that you get distracted more at certain times of the day, avoid tasks that require a great deal of attention at those times.

I was driving to an event in rush hour traffic through downtown Washington, D.C. I found myself jammed in the inner lane of a traffic circle when an ambulance got stuck about 75 feet behind me. I didn't know what to do—should I try to move forward to make space or move over to the side?

My bigger problem was that it was nighttime and my meds had run their course. I kept turning my head over my shoulder and watching the bright lights of the ambulance. I couldn't keep my eyes on the road ahead of me, even though I knew I should, even though I was trying. The siren kept calling me and the flashing lights kept mesmerizing me as I inched the car forward.

Luckily I didn't cause an accident.

Be aware of stimulus later in the day when you are tired, especially if you take meds and they have likely worn off. I am more easily distracted the later it gets in the day. I also find it harder to focus my attention on less dramatic tasks and things that I am not intrinsically interested in.

I know others who are affected by ADHD get more energized as the day goes on. I see those clients later in the day because they energize me due to the fact that I am intrinsically interested in them, especially as compared to paper work.

Need to Make a Plan!

Bottom line, when you are overwhelmed and trying to simplify your daily life, the thing to do is make a plan. The first step in making a plan is to get your head clear. A clear head makes for better decisions and planning.

To clear my head, I need to go to my organizer or planning calendar—a.k.a. "The Book"—and write down all the things I am trying to remember that I need to do this week. Next, I make a quick action plan for what is left to do on my project. Then I think only about knocking off the first thing on the action plan list. I don't worry about the rest but just focus on the first thing.

Finally remember: all you can do is what you have time to do. Worrying about how much time you have won't get you anywhere except using up some of that time. Too often because of ADHD we think of more complicated and difficult ways to do things than are really necessary. If we cut through the complications and difficulties, we are more likely to sustain the effort. If we are able to sustain the routine it will become a habit and we will simplify daily life.

Forget Perfect

De-cluttering your space is the first and best move toward simplifying your daily life.

The more paper you toss, the easier it gets. Become a paper tosser!

Simple systems are the ones you're most likely to follow.

A launching pad will make getting out of the door much easier.

Set up weekly and monthly charts with those tasks that you need to do regularly.

Chapter Seven

Communicating

Communicating poses particular challenges for those of us affected by ADHD. We tend to give too much information and over-explain, and we are often seen as making too many excuses. On top of that, we worry about doing things right and that gets in the way of listening to others. This chapter looks at how to avoid difficulties we have with communication, particularly over-communicating. It also talks about some ways that couples can communicate more effectively. For more help on communicating at work, also see Chapter 10: Working.

Lose the Preamble

When communicating with others, especially when explaining or answering questions about a project or task, people affected by ADHD tend to start by setting the scene. I call this the preamble. As in the preamble of the Constitution, we are situating our audience, letting them know our mindset and our thinking before giving the answer or explanation. This is something we need to lose.

When someone asks me how I became an ADHD coach, the direct answer would be to say that I trained as a coach, have ADHD, and found out that ADHD coaching is an actual niche and went for it. Instead, that ADHD brain of mine offers this answer: "Well I used to be a dancer, had this studio, and was a member of the dance company when I had one too many back injuries and had to get surgery, which was a failure. I ended up disabled and had to find a new career that I could work from home...."

Much of what I'm saying is unnecessary. I am creating a context for my answer that, in 90% of situations, is not necessary.

I believe the majority of us with ADHD are storytellers at heart so it is hard for us to communicate our thoughts and ideas without telling a story or giving some sort of preamble.

Keeping Communication Simple
If the answer to a question is 42, we want to set it up with what kind of 42 (Roman numerals or Arabic?) it is going to be and most likely how we decided and how we got there. Just say 42 and leave it at that.

The problem with preambles and superfluous storytelling is that you often lose your audience. They either drift away and stop paying attention or you find that you are cut out of the group. This can be a subtle process, but all of the sudden you realize that people are not calling you to go out or you're not being invited to group get-togethers. At work it may mean that you are isolated because people don't have time to interact with you or you are not picked for certain assignments because your boss cannot count on you to be succinct. This communication issue could hold you back both professionally and in personal relationships.

Ways to Speak Directly

> How long does it take to get to my mother's house? Short answer: 15 to 20 minutes. My answer: "Well, on a Friday afternoon before a 3-day weekend it can take 30 minutes. Of course, sometimes when it rains it can take even longer. And I remember when there was a hailstorm…"

If you feel you need to give some contextual information to help move the discussion forward or for someone to understand you, do it as concisely as possible. Hit only the most pertinent facts. Here are some ways to remind yourself to speak succinctly and get to the point.

Do the Preamble in Your Head

Try doing the preamble in your head and then just give a succinct answer. This takes practice. Another way to think about it is to give the bones without the flesh. Before I speak, I ask myself, "What are the bones?"

Question Yourself Before Speaking

Since not everything we think needs to be said aloud, one of my clients says to himself: Does it need to be said, and does it need to be said now? The fact is we often say too much and may say things that get us into trouble. These questions help us avoid creating potentially difficult situations due to speaking without thinking.

Be a Paramedic

Think of yourself as a paramedic rushing to hand off a critical patient in an emergency room. Before the paramedic speaks, the doctor or nurse asks, "What have you got for me?" That is, *Brief me on this patient's condition*. The key word here is *brief*. The paramedic gives only the critical facts as quickly and concisely as possible because time is essential to the patient's survival.

Thinking like a paramedic helps you to do two things:

1. Wait to be asked for introductory information. If not asked, don't give it.
2. If asked to give contextual information, give it concisely, and give only the information that is necessary.

Channel Joe Friday

Another way to get to the point is to think about the old Dragnet show where Sergeant Joe Friday says, "Just the facts ma'am, only the facts." I often repeat this to myself before I speak.

Ask If More Information Is Needed

The only contextual information you need to give is information that is vital to your audience's understanding. Sometimes I will give the short answer and then ask a question like, "Do you need any background information or a more detailed explanation?" This lets your audience decide if they want you to elaborate. If I am deciding, I will almost always choose to elaborate—whether it is necessary or not.

Stop Making Excuses and Giving Long Explanations

Many of us who have ADHD fall short of the mark sometimes. We deliver projects late, are late for appointments, fail to follow through, or forget something. This is part and parcel of being affected by ADHD. As a result, we get in the habit of rolling out explanations as to why we were late, didn't finish an assignment on time, didn't follow through, etc.

What sounds like an explanation to us sounds like excuses to non-ADHD people. After awhile they get tired of hearing our explanations so we need to stop giving them. Just say: *"Sorry, I am late."*

Not: *"I know I'm late, but you won't believe what happened while I was driving here. First a dump truck was ahead of me on a narrow street and I couldn't pass, then I had to rescue a kitty that was stuck in a tree, then I couldn't find parking...."*

Sometimes the reason we provide is true, and other times there is a little exaggeration. We are all guilty of it because the real explanation is embarrassing. "Sorry I didn't get it done. I know I had the whole weekend, but I was busy laying on my bed staring at the ceiling."

What sounds like explaining to us sounds like excuses to non-ADHD people.

It is better not to offer an explanation unless asked. Simply apologize and move on. If it is a work situation, get going on what is next, or get to work on what you were expected to have done.

The more we say, the bigger deal it becomes and the more likely it is that our transgression will be remembered. Keep your message short and sweet and most people forget. Save the explanation for those once-in-a-lifetime situations.

Part of the reason we over explain or even feel the need to explain at all is that we think somehow we need to justify ourselves. We are fearful of being viewed as less than or wrong, a thought that is almost unbearable. We so want to be believed. And that is where the irony comes in. The more we justify, the less likely we will be believed and the more likely the other person is thinking: Here he goes again! Why doesn't he just say he didn't get it done and get to work on it?

In answering the question, "Did you get the project done?" A "but" typically follows your answer: "No, but I have a really good reason. It all began on Wednesday when to my surprise a gorilla rang my doorbell..."

Instead, simply say, "No, I apologize. Is it possible for me to get it to you by the end of the day?" Then stop and listen.

Instead of Making an Excuse...

ACKNOWLEDGE

APOLOGIZE

OFFER REMEDY (if available) or MOVE ON (don't dwell)

The formula I have suggested is the best way to start breaking the justification habit. Use it until you find your own way of taking responsibility without giving laborious responses. Remember those explanations are not really for the listener's benefit but for our sensitivity of feeling less than in the eyes of others.

Each person must find their own language and decide what and how they want to take responsibility for their actions or lack of actions. "I messed up and now I am going to fix it." No prevarications. Take responsibility and remedy it. It is bold, mature, and shows self-confidence.

I seek this in my own actions. When I fail I simply get up off the floor and try to do better when the next opportunity presents itself.

Think Before You Disclose You Have ADHD

Another area you may be tempted to over-explain or "share too much" is around communicating that you have ADHD. My advice is to think twice before you disclose that you have a disability, even though certain things are hard for you.

I often remind myself, *Yes, I have a disability. But that doesn't mean I'm not able and not capable.* Despite the temptation to let everyone know about my ADHD diagnosis, more often than not I find that just moving forward is the best way to act.

> *I told someone that what they were asking me to do was difficult and that's why I was doing it slowly. His response: "You're only limited by what you think you can't do."*
>
> *It made me mad. I knew the reason I was slow was because of my learning disabilities, including slow processing in many different areas. I was definitely in one of those areas!*
>
> *I felt I had a legitimate excuse. I wanted to tell him…then I realized I was going to be slow with or without the excuse. Bringing up the excuse would have been for me, not for him. I still had to do what he was asking. I could have made him more sympathetic by pulling the disability card or I could just keep going at my pace and let him think whatever he would think of me. I chose the latter route because I am not responsible for others' opinions of me and I don't have to spend energy trying to control them.*
>
> *At the end he said how good it was that I kept on pushing forward despite how long it took—not, "God, you were so slow!" There was even a gleam of respect in his eyes. People pick up the energy of a trooper and remember that.*

Before you disclose that you have ADHD, think and ask yourself: Is it really going to help me in this situation? Will I earn more respect by simply pushing through and letting people pick things up through observation?

We have to be especially careful here since our explanations will likely be heard as excuses. It may not be fair, but as the saying goes, life isn't fair.

My advice is to pull out the big guns only when you absolutely need to. The feeling of satisfaction that you pulled something off in spite of the challenges you face every day is a true boost to your self-confidence. You'll feel on top of the world, being all that you can be.

You and the ADA

According to the Americans with Disabilities Act (ADA), you have a right to disclose your ADHD and not be discriminated against. Unfortunately not everyone believes that ADHD is real, and many coaches agree that unless you cannot get the accommodation in some other way, that it's better not to disclose. For example, if you are working in an open office and therefore are having trouble focusing, you might ask your supervisor if you can use a conference room to work in when it's not in use.

Dealing with Feedback

What happens when you fall short? (All of us do at some point—whether ADHD or not.) It's likely that you will hear about it. Learning how to listen to and respond to feedback is important.

Realize that feedback is often only given to people who are seen as having potential. Feedback indicates that someone (your boss, a co-worker) is willing to invest the time and effort in you. They may even be pushing for you to succeed. For example, when I was dancing, if you were corrected that meant the teacher saw that you had the ability to improve. If you make a shift and see feedback as just such an opportunity, other opportunities will open for you as well.

While some people can take feedback and let it roll off their backs, that is typically not the case for those of us with ADHD. We have difficulty receiving feedback from others, particularly if it's not 100% positive.

The reality is that there are times we mess up, fall down, and need help—and we're going to hear about it from other people, whether it's to offer help, correction, or advice. That's part of life.

Take the help, don't bristle at it. Hear what someone has to say about you and don't take it personally.

We need to learn to become a bit more receptive to this feedback. This is difficult for us. We are very sensitive to feedback that we deem is not absolutely positive. We see it as an attack on our person, not on our actions or our behaviors.

We hear: *bad person*. Not: *Would you like some help getting that project organized?* or *maybe you should start now because it tends to take you a long time to get things like this done.*

We hear: *You are a loser, a bad person*. We think: *She is always ragging on me, leave me alone. I always get it done...eventually.*

It is important to see that our actions or inactions impact others. So take the help, don't bristle at it. Hear the feedback and don't take it personally. Let it slide over you. Most people are trying to be helpful. They may not realize that how they present it to you does not always feel helpful to you. Just hear what someone has to say and move on. Do your best, that is all anyone can ask, yourself included.

Couples' Communications

Being in a relationship where one or both people have ADHD presents particular difficulties with communication.

Having Conversations That Stick

Partners of people affected by ADHD may have what they think is a good conversation with their partner, only to discover a day or two later that whatever was discussed is all but forgotten. This is not deliberate on the part of the person affected with ADHD. Nonetheless it is extremely frustrating to the person without ADHD, no matter how understanding they are.

What can be done about this? The following is a technique to improve the odds that a conversation has more of an impact in the moment, creates a lasting impression, and leads to a better understanding of what is being said by each party. This process is more formal and deliberate than a typical conversation. It also takes patience, something not always in great supply for people affected by ADHD.

Step 1: Each partner should think carefully about what they want to say and even make some notes if that helps to focus. Once the couple chooses who is going to go first, that partner makes one point, comment, or asks a question they wish to address. Be sure that it is just one.

Step 2: The second person then repeats back that point, comment, or question using their own words. This shows that the person is processing the information. The first person should not interrupt while the second person is reframing what they have heard. Then the first person comments as to whether the second person got the reframing correct. If not, the first person repeats what they want to communicate again, and the second person tries reframing again.

Stick with one idea at a time until both people feel as if they understand each other's point. This does not mean agreeing on everything, just that both partners feel they have been heard.

The conversation proceeds in this manner, point by point, issue by issue, until it comes to a conclusion. If necessary, take breaks (this is especially helpful for the ADHD partner). During those breaks no one is allowed to sneak in comments regarding the topic under conversation. The goal is to build respectful communication, and sideways comments will surely end that.

The best chance for couples to come to agreements is through this kind of a structured process, which facilitates real listening. Once couples come to an agreement, they may also write down their decisions to help both of them remember what it is.

Getting Your Partner's Attention

When a person affected by ADHD is focused on something, don't try and talk to them about another topic because most likely they won't remember it. If you need to get your partner's attention, one way to increase the chances of communicating effectively is through the eyes and maybe a little touch. Eye contact and entering the space of the person with ADHD make it more likely that the communication will stick. Consider these two scenarios:

Scenario 1

ADHD husband is sitting at the computer surfing the net. Wife calls out to husband, "Honey, don't forget you need to pick up Poopsy and Muffie from school in fifteen minutes."

No response.

"Honey," wife says an hour later (putting her hand on his shoulder), "Where are little Poopsy and Muffie?"

ADHD husband says, "Did you say something?"

Scenario 2

ADHD husband is sitting at the computer surfing the net. Wife comes up to husband, puts her hand on his shoulder, and says, "Honey, look at me. I need your attention." Then she waits patiently.

After a moment, she says. "Honey, I need your attention now. Look at me."

Husband looks up and she makes eye contact and holds the eye contact while she says, "Can you leave now and pick up Poopsy and Muffie from school? I know you don't want them to have to wait for you. You have been doing a great job this week with that. I appreciate it and I know they do too."

Couples often get into heated discussions about the person with ADHD not listening. Increase the odds of successful communication by stopping, getting in each other's space and making eye contact. (Know that these scenarios are not gender specific but ADHD specific!)

Forget Perfect

Make your explanations clear and succinct, not perfectly detailed or preambled!

Acknowledge, apologize, and move on.

There's no need to justify yourself.

Stick to making one point at a time with a person who is affected by ADHD and don't move until you know that person understands.

Eye contact and a little bit of touch can help get the attention of someone with ADHD.

Chapter Eight

Relationships

In life we have relationships with many people, and making them work makes life a lot better. This chapter deals with how to build friendships, develop relationships with family, and improve relationships as part of a couple. It also addresses the ongoing relationship we have with ourselves. In all of these relationships, we must value one another and ourselves, be open to changing how we relate to others, and, yes, forget perfect!

Valuing Yourself

I am listening to my family working on The New York Times Friday Crossword Puzzle. Friday's is always the hardest of the week.

It is amazing that we are together, my mom, brother, and nephew. My brother and nephew live in England so we rarely see them. The three of them are working away. My nephew is providing some of the answers. He is 11 years old! It is scary. I have no clue how I am related to this family. I am bad at crossword puzzles. They even do the puzzle in ink!

We all have different roles to play within our families, our communities, and the world at large. ADHD can sometimes make you feel apart from others, even your family. When you are feeling this, remind yourself of your worth and what you add to the mix. What are you good at? How do you contribute to either your family or the world? Maybe you are the spice!

Whether or not you have ADHD, we all forget to celebrate our uniqueness, especially when our lives are not going so well. It is crucial to double-down on celebrating who we are as individuals during troublesome times. Instead of getting hung up on all we can't do or have trouble doing, try to appreciate who we are. Forget measuring ourselves against other people. Forget perfect!

There will be some self-naysayers, those of us who tell ourselves that we haven't done anything special. Yet our existence alone has changed someone at some time. Think of what little or big thing you have done that has made a difference in another's life. If you can't think of anything, go do something:

- *Bake something and give it to a neighbor for no reason.*
- *Call a relative who isn't usually remembered.*
- *Mow an elder person's grass.*
- *Email a friend with a great book suggestion.*

It will make you feel great about yourself and will become the gift that keeps on giving because you are building relationships with others.

Building Relationships with Others

Developing friendships provides you with support in this world. If you are affected by ADHD, you may find that you have more challenges than others in developing those relationships. But you can surround yourself with those who value and support you which will greatly enrich your life.

Surrounding Yourself with Those Who Value You

I have a friend who always makes me feel special when we talk or see each other. She appreciates me and what I am doing professionally and personally. And here is the amazing thing—she tells me, not just thinks it. It is a great lesson.

We often think good things about friends and other people, but we rarely voice those thoughts to those people directly and in the moment. My friend says how she feels in the moment due to her positive nature. It is great to hear. Even when she disagrees with me, it is with such sincerity and desire to move toward understanding that I feel invigorated instead of feeling defensive.

Do your friends make you feel appreciated? Do you get off the phone feeling good about yourself? So often we stay in relationships that we haven't evaluated, and later find are really pulling us down.

When you are with a true friend, each parting feels like the gift of a new day. In other words, you have a feeling of hope, not doubt about yourself.

Be vigilant about the kind of friendships and the kind of friends you have. Create and nurture friendships that make you feel good, and gradually weed out the friends that make you feel less than. (This weeding out process can be done subtly.) These kinds of friends are not worth it and can do too much damage to your self-esteem. Friendship is an area where quality trumps quantity.

Expanding Your Circle of Friends

Making and keeping friends can be hard for people with ADHD for many reasons. These include a tendency to interrupt when others are speaking, lack of follow-up or follow-through, constantly being late, inability to provide undivided attention to another person, and having co-morbidities such as depression or OCD (obsessive-compulsive disorder).

When you are with a true friend, you have a feeling of hope, not doubt about yourself.

To meet new people, push yourself to get involved with activities that play to your strengths. If after you get to know somebody a problem such as your being late arises, apologize and together seek compromises that play to your assets, not your weaknesses. Don't make promises you can't possibly keep, like *I will never be late again.* One example of a good compromise is to have your friend call to remind you when to leave for an activity together. Your part is to thank them for the call and leave immediately.

A coach can help you move from the meet and greet stage to the friendship stage in a smooth and easy manner. Sometimes we ADHD people barrel right in when a more circumspect approach would be the better. For example, maybe you meet someone the first time you go to a Meetup and you've talked to them for 5 minutes, observed them during the meeting, offered to give them a ride home, and then tried to pin them down on plans for the next day.

Then there are those of us that can be antisocial. Learn to be more social. Think of developing a social life as planting seeds and growing a garden. It takes time, and you need to cultivate it so it grows. A coach can help you brainstorm what activities you might get involved in to meet other people and what to do if issues arise.

If you have hyperactivity that plays out verbally, you can go from interesting and exciting to annoying and overwhelming quickly. I used to be this person in certain situations. Luckily now it happens only rarely.

An example of such a scenario would play out like this:

> *You have the opportunity to meet a new group of people and you are excited because the theme of the gathering is something you know a lot about. This increases the likelihood that the people attending are your type of people. Even though it is hard for you to meet new people, you get over not wanting to go and get kind of excited about the gathering. Before you go, you remind yourself not to talk too much.*
>
> *At the event a few people introduce themselves to you. You're thankful because it is hard for you to initiate meeting new people. Then the group gathers for a short presentation and a discussion. You make a comment that is informative and witty. People look at you, smile, nod, and make follow-up comments. As the conversation continues, you notice that some information you believe is important hasn't been brought up yet. Not wanting to forget what you are thinking, you jump into the conversation and begin to monologue. The leader tries to gently get the conversation going again back to a dialogue. You jump in again, at times even interrupting people or trying to talk over them.*
>
> *You realize at some point that you need to pull back but for some reason you can't. When you first came to the gathering and made a few choice comments people were attracted to you. As you began overwhelming everyone, the early positive impression you made evaporates.*

You go home feeling depressed and mad at yourself, knowing that those few people you met at the beginning of the gathering whom you impressed were not likely impressed by the end of the evening.

Building Credibility

Another way to build relationships is by building our credibility with the people in our lives. What is credibility? It's the quality of being trusted and believed in. According to the dictionary, synonyms are trustworthiness, reliability, dependability, and integrity. We communicate this through our interactions with people in our lives.

Being someone who can be trusted to do what they say and is reliable can grease the wheels of life. It makes everything a little easier. With it, people cut you some slack. Without it, it is more difficult to recover from your mistakes.

Everyone has two credibility banks, one is a professional and the other personal. Both bank balances are extremely important. If either or both balances are low, our lives become trickier—we have no wiggle room—whereas a high balance in our bank gives us room to maneuver with people when we need to do so.

We always need to be building our credibility balance. In our personal banks we have multiple accounts such as:

- *Family*
- *Romantic partner*
- *Children*
- *Friends*
- *Relatives*
- *Neighbors*
- *People we do our personal business with such as doctors, lawyers, dry cleaners, pharmacists, plumber, banker*

We are involved with some people on a daily basis; with others, we have occasional interactions. In any case, it is important to have credibility with all the people who are important in your life.

Simply meeting basic expectations does not give you wiggle room. If you go the extra mile you will build up your different accounts, which will help you when something goes wrong or you need a favor.

> *I had to have some unexpected dental work done a few weeks after I had seen my dentist for my regular check-up. I didn't have all the money to pay for the unexpected work up front. My family and I had gone to this dentist and his father for years. I always paid my bills on time. For these reasons, I had credibility. When I asked if I could delay payment, there was no problem.*

Another instance of how credibility works is what I did with my inheritance:

> *I received an inheritance. The money arrived at just the right time because my old car was kaput. I bought a used car and thought about what to do with the rest of the money. I decided to give half of it to my brother. Years ago he had made it possible for me to move into my condo and he did so without expectation of getting any money back. Due to my disabilities it wasn't clear if I'd ever be able to work and he was very concerned about how and where I was living. Even though he had an inheritance coming too, I wanted to tangibly show my appreciation.*

What built my credibility in my brother's eyes was not the actual money but the fact that I didn't have to give it to him. He never asked for it, and he knew I could use that money. My giving him a chunk of it was a way of saying that I respected him and the sacrifice he had made for me.

Being in a Couples Relationship[9]

What happens when two people affected by ADHD get together in a relationship? Is it any different than when an ADHDer and non-ADHDer[10] get together?

Many of the issues are similar.

Addressing Problems of an Unequal Relationship

Usually one person is more affected by ADHD than the other. The less affected partner takes on the role usually played by the non-ADHDer in a relationship: the role of de facto parent.

The de facto parent role happens because it appears to the non-ADHDer that the ADHDer is not carrying their weight in the relationship. The non-ADHDer feels they have to take control or become the responsible one in the relationship.

One of the first things to go is the intimacy the couple once shared. Being cast in these new roles will diminish the sexual pull that the couple felt as romantic partners courting each other. Another way to think about this is one partner will begin to feel like a constant nag while the other partner begins to feel constantly badgered. Neither one feels good in the role they feel they have been forced into.

The situation that develops is no one's fault. The only fault would be if both partners were unwilling to realize that they each needed to make changes and modifications in their behaviors for the relationship to thrive.

Most often it is the non-ADHD partner who calls me about coaching their spouse to improve their marriage. One of the first things I ask is if they want their ADHD

9. Authors to check out on ADHD and relationships include Melissa Orlov and Gina Pera. I suggest initially reading Orlov's first book, *The ADHD Effect on Marriage: Understand and Rebuild Your Relationship in Six Steps.* It is a good introduction to the common traps ADHD couples fall into.

10. Here I refer to the partner not affected by ADHD as the non-ADHDer and the partner affected by ADHD as the ADHDer. While I dislike these terms because that person is more than just their ADHD, it makes delineations clearer when discussing couples affected by ADHD.

spouse to change some of his or her behaviors. The answer is always a big YES! Then I ask them the question that will decide if I take them on as clients: Are *you* willing to make changes in your behavior also? If I hear a yes, all systems are go. If I hear, "I don't need to make any changes, I am not the one with ADHD," all systems stop. I don't take them on as clients. Change is a catalyst for more change. If one person is changing their behavior and the other person isn't, there is no incentive to keep trying to change.

Additional Challenges for ADHD Couples

When one or both of the partners is affected by ADHD, there are additional challenges in the relationship.

Poor Memory

People affected by ADHD have an especially poor memory for conversations—especially if the ADHD affected person was doing something else during the conversation. The non-ADHD partner takes it personally that the conversation is forgotten. It feels like you don't care! In reality it is the ADHD at work.

The good news is that you can improve the odds that you will remember a conversation. Try these tips:

- *Stop whatever you are doing when you are spoken to so that you can listen.*
- *Take notes that you can refer to in your cell phone, on your calendar, etc.*
- *Ask your partner to repeat what was said if you are not sure what you heard a moment ago.*
- *Reframe, meaning repeat back what was said by your partner to them in your own words. Ask, "Did I get that right?"*
- *Apologize when you mess up. Don't make an excuse, just say, "I'm sorry, dear. I'll keep working on this. Remember this isn't about how important you are to me in my life."*

Impulsivity

People with ADHD often are impulsive. This can manifest itself in purchases that are not planned or discussed as a couple.

> "Honey, I got us a great deal on a house on my way home from work! Trust me, a little work and it will be worth twice what we paid!"

"Honey, while I was picking up the milk, I also picked up a new car! It's sweet!"

Similar unplanned, impulsive, or out-of-the-blue purchases can hurt a couple's relationship. A big financial expenditure may even put the couple in financial jeopardy. Keep in mind that the number one reason people get divorced is over money. Here are some approaches to dealing with impulsivity, yours or the other person's:

- *Wait 24 hours and then go back to see if you still want to buy it*
- *Discuss making a rule that the one person has to call the other before making a purchase, or over X amount that you must buy it together*
- *Ask these questions:*
    - *Do we need this or just want this?*
    - *Is there a place for it at home?*
    - *What will we get rid of in exchange for getting this?*
    - *Can we afford this?*
    - *Where else could the money go?*
    - *Are we saving for something and is that more important than this?*

Adjusting after the Honeymoon

A startling thing happens after getting married to those affected by ADHD. They change.

If it is the man who has the ADHD, which is statistically more likely, he will be Prince Charming during courtship, every woman's dream. They will do exciting things together. He will be attentive. He is in hunter mode. The ADHD-affected person is very stimulated during this part of the relationship. People affected by ADHD like novelty, so a new person in their life and a developing relationship is exciting. The unknown makes it attractive.

Then the ADHD man proposes, the couple marries, and things begin to change. The charming person who swept the woman away begins to disappear, replaced by someone who is easily distracted, who gets wrapped up in new things and new ideas, and who is on the computer for long periods of time.

This husband forgets things that he is told. He is often late. He is impulsive. He makes decisions without consulting his wife. He may even have difficulty holding down a job.

These things were not apparent when they were courting. How can that be? And what can you do about it?

People affected by ADHD can be adrenalin junkies. Once they have climbed Mt. Everest, the high is over. It is not that they were being inauthentic prior to marriage. The charmer is a true part of them, but not the whole of them. It is the stimulated part. Once settled into marriage they find it hard to keep that high going every day with regards to their spouse. In addition other parts of their personality begin to appear that may not be as attractive.

This can be incredibly shocking for the non-ADHD spouse. She thought she was marrying one man and she feels she got another. She is dismayed. She feels rejected. The level of attention she has been used to is gone. What is it she has done wrong? How can she fix it?

Here is where the real work of the marriage comes in. The couple will need to work hard to keep their marriage stimulating. Additionally, they each will have to adjust to this new reality. She will have to learn it is not personal when he is distracted, and he will have to learn to be sensitive to her need for him to be fully present when they are talking. It will take vigilance on both their parts, but improvement is possible. ADHD and marriage is hard but it can be rewarding.

Plan Spontaneity

This may sound contradictory, but planning spontaneity is important.

Don't make a specific plan but do schedule times for the two of you to do something special. This does not include staying in and watching TV. Nor does it mean buying tickets in advance for a play.

This is a time when you brainstorm as a team and come up with something new to do that is of interest or curiosity to *both of you*. No compromising by one to placate the other. You are a team solving an intriguing problem and then acting on it.

Why is it important to do this? Novelty is important to many people affected by ADHD. Plus, in most relationships there is usually a leader and a follower. This joint activity levels the playing field so that no one person is doing all the bending.

When Your ADHD Partner Refuses Medication

Medication can be an important part of a multimodal treatment for ADHD. While it does not work for all people affected by ADHD, it works for about 70% of them. Despite its effectiveness, some people don't want to take medication for ADHD. They think that ADHD and its effects only affects them and should be their personal choice.

But what if the person affected by ADHD is a part of a couple, even a couple with children? Is taking medication just a personal choice then? Should other members of the family or the other partner have input?

People affected by ADHD do not live in isolation. Should this make any difference in a decision about whether or not to take ADHD medication? I argue *yes*. When you are part of a team your actions affect the rest of the team. If you are playing first base in a baseball game, it is important to pay attention. If you were having trouble doing that, it would not only affect you but also your team's success.

People affected by ADHD often don't consider how taking meds (if meds work for them) can make a difference for others in the family. It could save a marriage. It could prevent disappointed kids. Children of parents with ADHD take their parents' behavior personally. They can't always rationalize that it was the ADHD acting and not the parent. For example, if they are constantly picking the children up late from school, it may be because of the ADHD. But children may interpret this as their parents not caring or remembering them.

If your partner refuses to even see if ADHD meds would work for them, explain how their actions or lack of actions make a difference in your relationship. Give specific, concrete examples. If you already know that ADHD meds work for them, try to find out why they won't take them and explain the consequences. Seek a compromise. Maybe they can take the stimulants just on the weekends. In any event, it is worth reopening the discussion when your ADHD partner refuses meds.

Dealing with Finances

Like many people with ADHD, do you often pay late fees on your bills even though you have the money to pay the bill at the time it is due? Have you gotten a ticket for not renewing your car registration on time even though you can do it online and you were sent a reminder?

You need help, especially if you are part of a couple.

You can automate some things, but some bills and obligations may not be regular enough or they require some scrutiny before being paid. But you don't, won't, or can't do it. Fortunately you can find help!

Hiring a Virtual Assistant (VA)

A VA is a virtual assistant you hire to take care of certain tasks for you. Generally you pay VAs hourly. They either work independently or for a company. You can search online for a VA or, if you know someone who owns their own business, ask them if they use and can recommend a VA.

Getting a VA may seem unnecessary, but it could save your relationship or marriage! Why? Because many couples affected by ADHD argue about chores. One of the most common difficulties is determining who is going to pay the bills, make

One of the most common difficulties is determining who is going to pay the bills, make appointments, and keep track of filings and registrations. Having a VA do it takes away the battle.

appointments, and keep track of filings and registrations. Having a VA take care of it not only takes away the battle but also the power issues that surround who manages the money day to day.

The big decisions can still be made jointly. The VA will just be directed on what to do. This reduces the possibility of the partner with ADHD acting impulsively or not at all. It also makes sure that the non-ADHD partner doesn't become the caretaker and master of the financial threads in the fabric of the partnership.

Barter, Trade, or Hire

Consider bartering, trading, or hiring out things that you dislike or have difficulty doing. I pay someone to do my taxes because I am not good at doing taxes. That doesn't mean I live in ignorance about them and abdicate all responsibility. I carefully chose my accountant. I am responsible for getting the proper information to my accountant in a timely manner, and have my taxes explained to me before I sign off on them.

In all areas of your life, take full responsibility. It can free you from uncomfortable obligations and help you become independent and empowered.

ADHD Couples Coaching

I coach ADHD couples all over the country, some in person and others over the phone. Sometimes I just coach a couple; other times I coach a couple and do individual coaching with each partner or one partner separately.

Usually it is the ADHD-affected partner who realizes the need for change from having heard it so many times from their non-ADHD partner. Sometimes it stems from threats such as, if you don't do something I am getting a divorce.

The non-ADHD partner usually wants the ADHD partner to lose their negative ADHD characteristics but remain the person they were originally attracted to. This can be problematic since sometimes ADHD characteristics were what attracted the partner in the first place.

Surprisingly it is not just the ADHD person who needs to adjust. As the saying goes, it takes two to tango. Both partners contribute to what is going on, so both of them need to make adjustments, not just the ADHD partner. This may be a shocker to the non-ADHD partner, who can be as resistant to change as the ADHD partner is.

Couples coaching is not the same as couples therapy. In coaching, every participant (coach and the partners) is considered an expert with a base of knowledge that contributes to solving problems. Unlike therapy, coaching does not deal with the psychological underpinnings of the relationship. Instead it emphasizes working on behaviors, such as changing communication styles and managing chores in a more equal way. ADHD coaching communicates an understanding of how symptoms of ADHD affect a relationship and, given those symptoms, finding strategies for improving the relationship.

Being Responsible for Yourself

In ADHD couple coaching, people tend to set up situations in their relationships that lead to failure. One such situation is asking the partner to be responsible for certain behaviors or actions. While this is important, it must be done with consideration.

Here's an example of how things get off the rails:

> *The non-ADHD spouse wants to lose weight so she asks the ADHD spouse to remind her each morning to go for a run and make sure she does it. This is bound to fail.*

First, we are each responsible for our own bodies. Second, you are asking your spouse to push you to do something you really don't want to do. Finally, you are asking someone who has trouble with memory and consistency to remember and be consistent—things that he has already frequently failed at.

This is a lose-lose-lose situation. She is going to be let down. He is going to feel guilty for not remembering, or resentful for having to take care of what's really her responsibility. Finally, she will not be able to lose weight, which was her goal.

In another situation, a non-ADHD spouse wants her husband to get up in the morning when she does for two reasons. First, so that he will exercise with her because she knows it will help his ADHD symptoms. Second, so that he will go to bed at the same time she does. She figures that if he has to get up earlier in the morning he will go to bed earlier. Like many people with ADHD though, he prefers to stay up late and has difficulty getting up in the morning. He is a night owl. She's trying to change that. He does try to go to bed early, but he lies in bed wide awake. The early bedtime doesn't work for him. It's not that he doesn't love her; it's simply not within his control. He is one of the many people affected by ADHD who have problems sleeping.

The value she placed on going to bed at the same time—early—conflicted with her husband's need to stay up late and his difficulty getting up early. He should be able to go to bed at the same time as proof of his love.

While it is fine to receive tips, pointers and even some help, those of us affected by ADHD must take full responsibility for our ADHD and not make others bear our issues. This means that you take responsibility for exercising, you figure out how to set up an alarm system to get yourself up in the morning, and you _______________ [fill in the blank]. These are your responsibilities, not someone else's.

Even though you are in a couple, ultimately you have to be responsible for yourself. To ask someone with whom you are in any sort a relationship to tell you what to do or tell you what to stop doing puts that person in a power position over you. This will affect your relationship and resentment may build on both sides due to the imbalance of power. And this is true for all relationships.

ADHD Parents with ADHD Children

Due to the heritability of ADHD, if you or your spouse has ADHD it is likely that your child will be affected by it as well. To help your child manage, you'll want to set up routines in your household that aid your child or children in developing their executive function skills. You'll then want to participate in some way with those routines as a family.

These can be routines to help your child finish their homework, get chores done, get in and out of the house with everything they need, and manage their room clutter. The list could go on.

Just as team members support their teammates, as a family you support one another around ADHD. After these routines have been successfully established and tweaked to work well for your child, it is time to integrate yourself and the rest of the family into those routines. In this way routines, which are necessary for everyone to function effectively, become a team effort. Having your family participate also allows your ADHD-affected child to no longer stand out as the one who needs the extra help. The reality is that you, and possibly others in your family, need structure too. When you all work on new habits and routines, your child isn't the only one getting extra reminders.

How does this work in practice?

One example is creating and posting a chart to help the ADHD child remember their household responsibilities. On this chart include all family members' responsibilities as well. This then becomes a reminder for the whole family and not just about "the one" with ADHD.

Those with "special needs," whether their disability is visible or invisible, are particularly sensitive to reminders and accommodations that others don't need. Making habits and reminders a family or team activity doesn't make the stigma go away completely, but it suggests that everyone needs a little support, and everyone makes mistakes and forgets things at times.

It may also help the ADHD child realize when they become an adult affected by ADHD that they are really not the odd man out. Everyone has something they are contending with, whether or not it is a "disability."

We do what is best for the team as a whole or the family as a whole. It can be lonely, embarrassing, and frustrating to be "the one" in the family, even if more than one of you is affected by ADHD. Make sure everyone in the family is on the same team. While each of you may be playing different positions or roles, this allows for dealing with ADHD to become a group effort. It also gives "the one" the opportunity to help his or her teammates, even if it is mommy or daddy. Actually it is more fun if it is mommy or daddy. And by becoming responsible for the other teammates "the one" learns that everyone in their family, on their team has their strengths and weaknesses. More important, the feeling of being singled out may diminish because they feel as if they are contributing to and supporting others on the team.

Forget Perfect

Make friends with people who appreciate you for who you are.

Get involved with activities that play to your strengths.

To make sure you're listening to and understanding the other person in a conversation, take notes!

ADHD or not, take responsibility for yourself.
Don't try to get others to get you to do what you need to do for yourself.

If meds are effective for you or your partner,
they can vastly improve your life and that of your family.

Chapter Nine

Career and Unemployment

Many who are affected by ADHD have difficulty being successful in their careers, particularly if they are working in a field or in a job that is not of interest to them. They are also more likely to face unemployment. This chapter provides strategies to deal with unemployment, find a job, and, most importantly, find work that you can be passionate about.

The first time I read Studs Terkel's book ***Working*** *I was in college studying oral histories of American labor history.* ***Working****, Terkel's best known book, is based on three years he spent talking with people in all sorts of occupations. The subtitle explains it all:* ***People Talk About What They Do All Day and How They Feel About What They Do.***

I have never forgotten a quote from the last page of the book's introduction. A woman named Nora Watson said, "I think most of us are looking for a calling, not a job. Most of us, like the assembly line worker, have jobs that are too small for our spirit. Jobs are not big enough for people."

Find a Career That Is a Calling

In my family, you didn't just have a job or a career, you had a calling. Your work was to fight for the good of others based on what you believed were inequalities in our society. Both my mother's and father's work (as advocate for gender equality and labor leader, respectively), though on the surface appearing to be different, were actually working toward the same goal and reflecting the same values. Both believed that people, no matter their gender, race, ethnicity, socio-economic background, occupation, or religion (LGBT issues weren't talked about back then), had a right to have a voice or representation at the table.

Growing up I simply assumed that everyone had a job that was about saving the world. (I don't know how I explained all the other people around me who worked making my life and the lives of others function, whether by driving a bus or umpiring a baseball game.) I also thought that you intrinsically knew what type of work you were meant to do. I thought everyone knew their "special how"—how they were going to change the world. How they in particular were meant to do it—be a doctor, a social worker, or a community organizer. Now as an adult I understand that we need people in all types of occupations to make society work.

If at all possible find your occupational calling. It will make your life easier.

I still believe if it is at all possible to follow a calling ,that you should, I also know that you don't need to be in a certain occupation in order to fulfill a calling. Your calling could be that as you interact with the public in whatever job you do, that you do it with heart. As a shoe salesperson, your calling could be to serve your customers to the best of your ability and with honesty and compassion.

I bet you have met people who leave you feeling better for having met them, even after just a brief interaction. So a calling can be a specific occupation or how you approach any occupation. But here comes my caveat: if at all possible I urge you to find your occupational calling. When all is said and done, it will make your life easier.

Play to Your Strengths, Not Your Weaknesses

If you're affected by ADHD you may find that you have taken on jobs or even lifelong careers that play to your weaknesses, where there was a high likelihood of failure. You may have done this for any number of reasons:

- *You believed it was a safer career choice than one of intrinsic interest.*
- *There were more jobs available with that particular career choice.*
- *The particular career paid better.*
- *There was pressure from family to have a prestigious occupation.*
- *What you are good at is not of value to society so you chose something society does value.*

If you have ADHD and choose a job or career that you are not inclined towards, it is less likely that you will able to hold that job or be successful in that career. Keep in mind that a higher paying job will not result in more money if you lose that job.

The flip side is that if you do something that is strength- or interest-based, you are more likely to be successful. A lower paying job that is right up your alley may result in more money because you are able to stick with it and move up in the organization or the profession.

Smart career choices are not clear cut. They depend on you—your interests, strengths, weaknesses, needs, and wants and how those intersect with opportunities and needs of society.

Know Your Strengths

A typical ADHD story is the long-time emergency room nurse who is great at her job. The powers that be promote her to head nurse supervisor. She's now responsible for scheduling the nurses, attending administrative meetings, tracking inventory, etc. There is no intensity or in-the-moment pressure. She starts to fail.

This woman, who is smart and knows herself, asks to be demoted, even though it means going back to her former pay grade. The emergency room is where she thrives and is a star. Quality of life is important and she knew that being miserable all day was not good for her.

(Adapted from Dr. Ned Hallowell, *Driven to Distraction.*)

Choose Intrinsic Interests

Those of us with ADHD tend to devalue jobs or tasks we are good at or that intrinsically interest us. We tend to see them as silly or unimportant. Conversely we put greater value on things that are hard for us or that we are not naturally inclined to do. For that reason people affected by ADHD pursue jobs that are very detailed oriented (for example, those requiring a lot of paperwork), when instead they could be seeking jobs that focus on idea generation, where someone else does the documentation. Above all, the job should be of intrinsic interest so that the person is motivated to succeed at the parts of the job that are difficult for them.

I had a framework that I used to use when I was teaching. I called it "challenging in a situation of success." It meant that it was important to challenge each student to reach as far as they could but not so far that there was a high likelihood of failure. It is good to be challenged. It is one of the ways we grow, but constant failure can be discouraging enough to paralyze a person.

People with ADHD who work in jobs or are in fields they are not passionate about make, I believe, a major mistake. It is hard enough for us to get things done when we are interested. Putting ourselves in a position of having to get things done when we are not interested seems to me to be ludicrous. I realize that sometimes we don't have a choice, but the goal should always be to move toward a career or job where there's a higher probability that we will do what we need to do to be successful. Without intrinsic interest it is much more difficult to start a task, finish a project, and move forward in our career.

In creating a positive life with ADHD, I strongly encourage you to seek a life where the scale is weighted heavily on the intrinsically interesting side. If you remove the intrinsically un-interesting as much as possible, you will find more success and peace.

If you have passion or are working towards a passion you are more likely to think, both on and off the job, about what needs to be done in a positive way. Your mind will be working away figuring things out. You will be:

- *Drawing up the best way to approach a task or project.*
- *Solving something that has you stymied.*
- *Identifying who might be good to work with or to whom to delegate what needs to be done.*
- *Figuring out a more efficient process.*
- *Determining how important something is and if you should continue doing it.*
- *Coming up with new ideas and connections that help move you forward.*

Many people struggle with finding their passion or intrinsic interest because they believe that they should have only one passion—and that passion should be obvious to them.

> *I started dancing at the age of five. When I was injured and could no longer dance or teach dance at age thirty, I thought I was destined to work in some other career that would be just a job to me. At the same time, I knew if I wasn't interested in what I did it would be hard to do the work. Luckily I discovered another passion: helping people affected by ADHD. At first it wasn't a passion, it was an interest. As I learned more and developed my skills, my passion grew.*

Today, because people usually live much longer than in the past, we tend to become an expert in more than one thing. Many of us have two, three, or more careers in our lifetime. It is possible to be passionate or intrinsically interested in each one of them.

It may require extra effort, some lean times, or a coach to find a career and job of great interest to you. But you spend a large chunk of your life working. Why not make it easier to do and more enjoyable?

Getting a Job After Losing One

People often seek coaching when they have been put on probation by their employer and are in a tough spot. Many times it is already too late to save their current jobs. Other times, the job is saved, but once that person is off probation they think they are in the clear and repeat the behavior that put them on probation in the first place. Then they quickly lose their job without notice.

Getting another job when you have a poor work history, especially if you have been fired, is not easy. The first step is to get over losing your job and make the decision to move forward. It is critical to make this transition quickly. Statistics show that the longer you are unemployed the less desirable you become to employers. They wonder why no one has hired you.

Applying for Jobs Immediately

People affected by ADHD are inclined to procrastinate in this type of situation. Granted, job hunting is not fun for most people, but the sooner you begin getting applications out there the greater likelihood you will get hired. Very few people get unsolicited job offers at the right moment in their lives. No applications sent means lower odds of getting a job.

The sooner you begin getting applications out the greater likelihood you will get hired.

One approach to get moving is to challenge yourself to see how fast you can collect 100 "No's." When applying for jobs, you are likely to get negative responses no matter what. This probability often gets in people's way. They are afraid of being turned down so they don't apply, or a rejection email or no response upsets them and they stop taking action.

Take this on directly. Challenge yourself by making your job-hunting process a quantitative exercise. It can take away some of the emotion and the fear of being turned down loses some of its power over you.

Sometimes I hand my client a page with 100 no's on it, or I have them make their own page. Then they apply to as many jobs of interest as they can find. The goal is to cross all the No's off the list as fast as possible because it's likely that by the time you get through 100 No's there is a Yes waiting. I have never had a client cross out all of the No's. Most usually get a job before they have crossed out even 30 No's. By taking away the fear of rejection, you focus your energy on applying for jobs.

Avoiding Job-Hunting Pitfalls

Most people search online when looking for a job. It is a great place to start, but I see the same mistakes made over and over again: limiting the job search to online listings, getting caught up in *looking* at job listings instead of *submitting* applications, and continually rewriting the cover letter.

Online Only Won't Cut It

The first mistake is to only look online for job opportunities. Roughly half of all available jobs are not listed and are found through other means such as networking. Yes, that means getting out there and talking with people. Many of us affected by ADHD do not like to do this. It ranks right up there with making phone calls as an activity we don't like to do. But it is a must if you want to find a job in a reasonable amount of time.

Keep Those Applications Moving

The second mistake is hoarding job listings. Instead of finding a good job possibility and then applying, the job seeker continues to look at listings for more jobs to apply for. The list gets longer and longer, then they never get around to applying for those jobs—they just read about them. Don't do this! If you find a listing or a job that you might like, read it carefully, and apply. Then start again. Do not pile up job descriptions to apply for later. Later often doesn't happen for those of us with ADHD!

Get the Cover Letter Done

The third mistake is writing and rewriting your basic cover letter and resume. Thinking that if you keep working on them you will hit some point of perfection is a form of procrastination. If you are rewriting, then you are not actually applying for jobs, and if you don't start applying you can't get rejected.

Here's where time can be your friend. Take 3 to 5 minutes and write the worst cover letter that you can. I'm not kidding. When the time is up, look at the letter. You'll find that there are always some good sentences hidden within this terrible cover letter. If in 5 minutes you can purposely write a terrible cover letter that has some good sentences, then it's more than likely you can write a good cover letter and be done with it within a half-hour or an hour.

Practice Interviewing

If you are not moving your job application process forward, it may be because you fear getting an interview and having to face questions you don't want to answer or don't know how to answer. If this sounds familiar, try role-plays and mock interviews that hit on the really tough questions you are worried about. Ask a friend to play the evil interviewer. Doing this many times will build your confidence to the point that it is unlikely you'll face a question that you haven't already practiced. If your friend becomes the truly evil interviewer, then the real interviews will be a piece of cake.

Finally, know that if your work history is not great, the quantity of applications is going to count. You will get better at talking to prospective employers with each interview you have. You will find ways to discuss the loss of your job or your poor work history, maybe even the lack of glowing recommendations. Practice and pressure will improve your job-hunting skills.

Consider Entrepreneurship

Many people with ADHD are successful in their own businesses, especially if they do something they love. They are more likely to get the work done and be passionate about what they are doing.

People with ADHD become entrepreneurs for a number of reasons, including:

- *They don't like having a boss or supervisor over them.*
- *They don't take critical feedback or evaluations well.*
- *They like being in charge.*
- *They believe being an entrepreneur will give them freedom to live the way they want.*
- *They believe they can make more money.*
- *They like to do things a certain way.*
- *They believe they have a great idea or service that they do particularly well.*
- *They like the excitement and stimulation that comes with getting a business started.*

If you are considering entrepreneurship, consider both the upsides and downsides before making a move.

Weighing the Pros and Cons

There are definitely both pros and cons involved in working for yourself instead of for someone else. Here's a good starting point when considering your options:

PRO	CON
In charge of self	In charge of self
No one telling you what to do	No one telling you what to do
Highly productive under pressure	Poor productivity without pressure
Big idea developer	Difficulty with small details
Set your own hours	No fixed work hours
You decide income	You have to earn income
No bureaucracy	No structure or systems in place

There are many successful ADHD entrepreneurs and, I am sure, more than triple that number of *unsuccessful* ADHD entrepreneurs. If you do decide to go this route, my best advice is that as soon as you start your business, take what little money you have and hire a virtual assistant to handle the details. It will be money well spent. You do the big idea stuff that brings in money and have the assistant take care of the details like invoicing, preparing bank deposits, keeping records of contacts, etc.

Setting Up a Business Partnership That Works

In my first business venture, I had a partner who knew more about business than I did. This helped me learn about what I would do and what I would not do if I ever went into business on my own. It was as if I played in the kiddie pool before diving into the grownups' pool. This was very helpful the second time around because I knew more about what I was getting into.

If you do decide to work in a partnership, the first step is to consider who you are partnering with and draw up a legal agreement that covers the contingencies for the many ways the partnership could change. This is definitely a relationship in which you need to look before you leap. Don't just start together impulsively as we ADHD folks tend to do.

Following your intrinsic interests will make it more likely that you will succeed at your work and be happy. By doing so, you may have to lose some of your beliefs about what work is valuable and important. Instead, consider that what is important is what you do well and easily.

Forget Perfect

Find a career that plays to your strengths, not your weaknesses.

Ask yourself, what's your passion?

If you've lost your job, start applying immediately and don't get hung up on writing the perfect resume and cover letter.

When it comes to getting a job, numbers (of applications) count.

Consider becoming an entrepreneur, and if you do, set yourself up to be successful.

Chapter Ten

Working

In many ways, the workplace is like a boot camp for people with ADHD. When you work for someone else, you need to be on time, not procrastinate, keep your work area uncluttered, set up systems that make you more efficient, respect the power of authority (your boss), follow the rules, learn to listen to feedback (some of it no doubt negative), and not make excuses. That's quite a list! While this all may seem daunting, know that what's expected of you at work is what's expected of everyone else. And working is how we earn a living to support ourselves and the life we desire. Especially if you are employed by someone other than yourself, you'll have to be alert to the numerous pitfalls that people with ADHD can encounter in the workplace. That is what this chapter is designed to help you with.

Problems People Affected by ADHD Face at Work

The day-in and day-out problems of ADHD can become magnified at work. Our weaknesses are often the basic, prized attributes of a good employee. Common issues that come up in the work environment for someone with ADHD are related to time management, organization, planning, relationships, and communication.

Being On Time

Being on time for work is a basic and reasonable expectation employers hold for their employees, yet it is hard for many people with ADHD to do.

Many people with ADHD try very hard to be on time but they find that more often than not they are late. Others don't even try to get to work on time. They have the attitude that as long as they get the work done, it shouldn't matter what time they get to work. Or they think if they stay late at work to make up the time, the slate is clean and their boss shouldn't have a problem.

This is just not true. It is reasonable for both bosses and colleagues to be upset when you are late all of the time. If your colleagues make it to work on time, in their minds it is not fair if you are not held to the same standard. And if you don't arrive when you are supposed to, you are not available to them or your boss. This can make it hard to get work done because in most workplaces completing work is a team effort.

Work the Hours You're Assigned

Many people with ADHD think that as long as they put in an 8-hour day it doesn't matter if they are late to work. They figure, well, I will just stay late. Same difference.

But in the employer's mind that is not true. If you are supposed to be at work from 9 a.m. to 5 p.m. Your boss wants you available during those hours. Working until 8 p.m. but being unavailable at 9 a.m. doesn't wash unless you have an agreement with your employer from the onset. As an employee you are at your job at the behest of your employer, not the other way around.

There are so many other things that we struggle with and have to overcome in our jobs that it is even more important that we follow the rules and requirements as closely as we can. Even if it is difficult, the most fundamental rule is getting to work on time.

Doing What You're Told

In general, people with ADHD don't like to be told what to do. A sense of resistance arises within them if direction isn't given in what they see as an appropriate manner. If this happens to you, it can cause problems at work. This is especially true if you are starting out in the workforce and are at the bottom of the power hierarchy. In that position, people are *always* telling you what to do.

Controlling Impulses

Impulse control can be another minefield for people with ADHD. The person with ADHD may spontaneously blurt out something inappropriate at work without thinking through the ramifications. It may be a remark aimed at a co-worker or a comment about the management that gets him or her in hot water.

People with ADHD may quit their job in the heat of the moment rather than taking a deep breath or some down time before addressing a burning issue they have with their superior.

Related to impulsivity is the tendency to give TMI (too much information) to co-workers. A classic example of TMI is revealing at work that you have ADHD. This can backfire on you. The person you told may not have a problem with your ADHD, but what if they tell a person in a position of power over you who has negative feelings about ADHD or thinks ADHD is a lazy person's excuse? Your career could be damaged.

So think twice about what you reveal at work. Assume everyone will know what you tell one person. Only tell your coworkers what you're willing for everyone to know.

Staying Motivated

Keeping motivated when you have tedious work to do is hard. Remember that tasks that seem insignificant contribute to the bigger picture. To prevent letting work slip through the crack, make lists and appointments with yourself so you make sure to complete the boring tasks that need to get done. I motivate myself by thinking how good I will feel when those tasks are completed. A coach also helps me to organize, prioritize, and set goals that keep me moving forward.

Not Making Excuses

Those of us with ADHD often find that if we have handed in work late, been late to a meeting, gotten to work late, or forgotten an appointment, we tend to offer excuses. In our minds we are explaining what happened, but the other party is thinking, "Here we go again...another long, drawn out excuse!"

Instead of offering excuses, simply apologize and either ask how to proceed or offer a possible solution to the problem. For example, "I apologize for not having the project done on time. Here is how I plan to get it done. I've included milestone dates in order to track my progress. Is this how you want me to proceed or do you want to handle this in a different way?"

It is hard to simply take responsibility for the end result without getting an opportunity to explain ourselves, but if we don't explain we gain more respect in the end.

Communicating at Work

Next time you are in a sticky situation, own up to it. Then show how you plan to solve it and ask if that is the route your boss wants you to go.

Instead of This:
"The project isn't done but you won't believe what happened when I was trying to work on the project. I got inundated with other work and on top of that I had the flu!"

Try This:
"I'm sorry. I can give you a written summary this afternoon so you can see just what I have finished and what still needs to be done. "

There is one caveat to this: if something significant happens that would foul up anyone, such as a death in the family, then speak up.

Channeling Adrenaline at Work

People with ADHD do well at work such as emergency medicine, sales, or fire fighting because they are at their best in high-pressure situations. A job with some sort of thrill factor helps many people with ADHD perform better.

But almost any kind of work has aspects that don't carry that thrill factor, and it is the mundane side of jobs that many people with ADHD find so difficult. They have trouble activating themselves to get things like monotonous paperwork done.

The key is to try to carry the momentum from the thrilling activities over to the not so thrilling activities. How do you do this? Sometimes the answer is to make a game of the activity or to time yourself.

Receiving Feedback

In most jobs, your performance is formally evaluated each year. If you happen to have a good manager, you will receive feedback day in and day out about what you are doing well and what you need to improve on but more often this feedback is less frequent.

Generally, people affected by ADHD do not take feedback well if there is any negativity, correction, or any call for improvement at all. When we get this feedback, we want to explain the circumstances beyond our control that made it difficult, if not impossible, to complete a project on time or perform at our best.

We may be overly sensitive because we have grown up being criticized or receiving back-handed compliments such as "You would do so well if you only applied yourself!" Whatever the reasons for this sensitivity, it is important to learn how to manage it better. I struggle with this myself. My advice is to receive the information for what it is—information. Distance yourself from it, and don't take it personally. This is not about you as a person but about your actions. If you can receive feedback this way, life will be a lot less stressful.

Consider Feedback as Information

One of the best responses to feedback on an action you need to change is simply to say, "Thank you. I will work on that." Even better, also write down the correction because it shows your supervisor that you are taking it seriously. If you want clarification or more specific information, ask, "Could you give me some examples of this behavior?"

Above all, instead of trying to prove the person wrong, show that you want to understand and improve. You can also get back to them with a plan to address the issues your supervisor feels need improvement. It will be impressive.

It may go against your instincts not to explain and give reasons for what you did, but explaining doesn't show you in the best light. Instead, let your actions speak. Remember it was your actions that made your supervisor come to the conclusions that led to the critique.

A Feedback Response Scenario

Those of us with ADHD have had so much failure in the past that we can be very sensitive to feedback. We may feel insecure about aspects of our work and take feedback as criticism. Aside from ways to respond that are discussed above, we also need to know how to shift what we feel and hear in situations like this.

> **First,** *breathe! Deeply, to relieve the tension that has developed in your body in reponse to the defensiveness we feel.*
>
> **Second,** *try to embrace the idea that this is not about who you are but about a product you are creating.*
>
> **Third,** *think of yourself as on the same team as the person giving you the feedback. Think of it as feedback not a critique. It is simply their opinion. You can take it or leave it.*
>
> **Finally,** *we can't be an expert in all things. So shore up your internal sense by reminding yourself of what you do know and can do well. Remember that this is an opportunity to hone another skill. So take a deep breath, relax, and be receptive to this person's expertise.*

All of this is hard, but feedback is a part of life. How you take it demonstrates your strength of self. It is you who chooses how the situation unfolds.

Building Professional Credibility

Each of us wants to build credibility in both our personal and professional lives. When we have credibility, we are given the benefit of the doubt and have more options. I liken this to having a bank account. When we build up money in our account, we have more flexibility in what we can do in our lives.

With respect to credibility, having a high balance in our credibility bank account changes how people treat you and what they will do for you. Let's imagine my professional credibility bank account was high because of 100 special favors I did for my boss. When I ask for Friday off, he is more likely to give it to me because the balance in my credibility bank is high.

Conversely, if I have been late to work often and am not getting my projects done on time, my professional credibility bank account's balance is probably low. So it is less likely I'll be granted my request. I haven't earned it. There is not a big enough balance to make a withdrawal, so it's likely I can't have the day off.

If you are always on time to work and finish your projects on time you might earn a little credibility to add to your bank account. But here is where many people with ADHD falter. They think that doing what's expected should earn them a lot of credibility. You are supposed to get to work and finish projects on time. That is the job. It doesn't matter that it takes extra effort for those of us affected by ADHD. However, if we arrive at work on time, get our projects in on time, *and* do something extra for the company or boss, then we earn extra credibility points. Our balance shoots up and it is more likely that we will be allowed to take off on a Friday.

It's good to be seen as a reliable employee, but going beyond basic expectations is what builds credibility. Don't misinterpret getting done what is required of you as something deserving of extra credit. Our struggle with getting what's expected done is really *our* problem. We will gain more respect if we just do the work and refrain from explaining why it is a big triumph when we are simply meeting the basic expectations.

You can choose how you will go beyond basic expectations. The smart way is to use your strengths and what is unique about you. Determine what you do well and how it fits in with your organization's goals. Then do something extra related to that if you want to earn credibility.

Working on Long-Term Projects

Another area of difficulty for people with ADHD is managing long-term projects. Prioritizing and managing time, setting milestones, estimating how long each task is going to take, and identifying the best process for completing each project can be difficult. These issues involve skills related to executive functions, which are markedly weaker for individuals with ADHD.

While the context here is projects at work, many of the same processes and pitfalls apply to long-term projects in other parts of your life.

If Nothing Is Said About the Project, It Still Exists

After you are first assigned a long-term project, you may not hear about it again from the person who assigned it to you. As a result, you may either forget about it, think it is no longer important, or think the person has forgotten about the project. The assumption might be, *If they aren't saying anything about it or coming to me for it, it probably isn't that important.* Wrong!

It is assumed that you are a responsible adult. You are expected to keep track of your own projects and get them in on time regardless of whether or not you are prompted or asked about the project.

Seeking Clarification and Avoiding Procrastination

If you are not sure how to start on a project or what to do, you may start to procrastinate. This procrastination can last so long that sometimes the project is never started or is started too late. For that reason, it is important to get the clarification you need up front so you have the information you need to do the work.

A common occurrence is waiting until late Friday to start a project due Monday. The ADHD mind thinks: I have two days to get this done. What the ADHD mind often doesn't anticipate is the need for key information over the weekend that another colleague has at the office. The project won't be completed in time and may disrupt the work of other people who were counting on the project being finished on Monday.

When we feel like putting things off, it is helpful to anticipate how not doing something might affect another person negatively.

Our actions and inactions often have ramifications for other people and ourselves. When we feel like putting things off, it is helpful to anticipate how not doing something might negatively affect another person. That other person may think less of you or no longer trust you with things that are important to them. Inaction could lead to loss of opportunity in the future.

Thinking about this often helps me get started on things I want to put off. For example, I don't like pursuing people for money owed me in my business but there are serious ramifications if I don't get that money. I won't be able to pay people I have hired and I won't be able to pay myself, which will result in bills going unpaid and services being stopped. Furthermore, if it goes on awhile, I would have to stop helping people affected by ADHD, something I feel is a calling, in order to find work that will provide me a paycheck. All this could happen just because I put off collecting money owed to me.

Always think through the implications of *not doing* something. It may help activate you.

Asking for Help

When those of us with ADHD get into muddles we are fearful to ask for help. Why don't we ask for help? Do we feel ashamed? Maybe all we need is to talk through the issue to become clearer on what the issue actually is.

If we wait, getting more stressed, we dig the hole deeper.

Instead of waiting until the clock has just about run out on us, try asking for help up front. It gives both the helper and us the opportunity to do something about the situation at hand.

We don't look down on other people who ask for help. And we're usually more than willing to offer our help. There's no reason to have this double standard. So just ask. Let people know what you need. You may be surprised at what you get back.

Chunking Out the Project and Plotting Your Time

When you are given a long-term project, first figure how to get from where you are starting to where you need to end up. One of the best ways to do that is called chunking. Chunking is dividing a project into manageable chunks or steps. Start by looking at due dates, and then back out the work from there.

This book, for example, started as a bunch of index cards. Each index card had on it a topic I wanted to cover in the book. The next chunk was putting the index cards in some sort of working order and creating an outline to give me a foundation. The next chunk was looking at my previous writings to see if I could match them to the outline. This would help me use material that I already had on hand. The next chunk was figuring out what still needed to be written. I think you get the idea.

The point is to figure out all the chunks of work or steps you need to go through before you start the project. Granted, you will likely find that during the project you missed some steps or that some of the steps you anticipated turned out to be unnecessary. Simply do the best you can to forecast what the chunks will be. Like a weather report, it will not be perfect but it will give you enough of an idea of how to proceed.

Do the best you can to forecast what the chunks will be. Like a weather report, it will not be perfect but it will give you an idea of how to proceed.

Once you have your chunks, estimate how much time each chunk will take. Look at the total time you have. If the time it takes to do each chunk is more time than is allocated to the project, then you will have to take action. You can clear time in your schedule, delegate tasks or chunks, or ask for more time to complete the project.

It is important to be realistic as to how long each step will take you. Those of us with ADHD are notoriously unrealistic about how much time tasks take us. It doesn't matter if they are little or big tasks. I like to think it is because we are optimists but somehow I suspect it really has to do with executive function issues.

Building Your Timeline

To build your timeline, you'll want to back out tasks from the end to the beginning. Backing out is taking the last chunk and putting it near (but not flush against) the end date. Then put the next to last chunk or step in front of the last chunk and so forth.

Once you have a timeline it is easier to start the tasks or chunks within the long-term project because they are broken down into bite-size pieces.

For instance, if this book was going to come out in December then that meant scheduling four weeks before December for the interior design and processing. Before that the book would have to be copy-edited, which would take maybe two weeks. Before that, the developmental editing and three drafts with rewriting. Backing all that out would mean I would have to have finished writing the first draft by the end of September or beginning of October. I would not have known that if I hadn't backed out all the chunks.

Chunking and time estimation helps you build a timeline for your project. Once you have a timeline it is easier to start the tasks or chunks within the long-term project because they are broken down into bite-sized pieces. These are easier to approach than looking at a big project. Looking at a big project, you often don't know where to start. Once it is broken down into bite-sized chunks it is much easier to attack because it is less intimidating to do an hour or a chunk a day than to get 8 hours of the project done in a single day.

Be aware that as you go you will be constantly adjusting your timeline because things happen. As it turned out, finishing the writing by September or early October wasn't enough time, so the backing out of the chucks had to be redone. Some things will take longer than you think and other things will take less time than you think.

Leaving Time to Check Your Work

Be sure to budget extra time at the end of the project to review and check your work for mistakes, typos, and errors. These things make a difference as to how people view your work and your capabilities.

Under Promise and Over Deliver

When you are planning a project, it is best to under promise and over deliver than the other way around. We are great idea generators and we sometimes get ourselves in trouble making a simple project more complicated than it needs to be. Get done what you were asked to do first and on time. If you have extra time then go the extra mile but not before you have gotten the required part done.

Avoid Taking Too Long to Get Projects Done

Unfortunately with ADHD we tend not to think ahead. We can get caught up in perfectionism and forgetting that done is better than, you guessed it—perfect. Each project or assignment we are given has a value or importance. Doing this kind of thinking helps us to know how long to spend on a project. If I spend all day on a project that will ultimately have little effect on my business in its longevity, prestige, client service, or fiscal stability, I have wasted a lot of time. The project only merited a short amount of my time. If the project would move my business substantially forward, it is worth devoting a substantial chunk of time to the project.

When working for others if you are not sure how long to spend on a project or you don't know the relative importance of it to the company—ask.

- *How much time were you looking for me to spend on this?*
- *Do you want a survey or an in-depth study?*

Be sure to ask the time-value ratio without devaluing or comparing it to other work. You never know what is someone's pet project and you don't want to make the mistake of comparing projects and be perceived of devaluing another project. If anyone is going to devalue a project, let that be your boss or supervisor, not you.

Avoiding Non-Work-Producing Activities

Be careful not to get hooked into doing non-work-producing activities. These are activities that circle around the work you need to do but don't bring you closer to the finish line. As people with ADHD, we are famous for doing this even as a deadline looms.

In writing this book I created a detailed outline of all the topics I wanted to cover. Then I looked at what I had already written and cut and pasted previous writing where it fit in the outline. Going through the document it was clear what topics I still needed to write about. I could simply have worked from the beginning of the document, filling in where nothing was written. Simple, right? Not for me! For each section I copied the topics I hadn't written on in my own handwriting on a piece of notebook paper. The paper then went into my official binder. When I was ready to write, I took the list and recopied it onto a white-

> *board so I could see where I was on my list without having to look at my binder or turn a page. When I completed a topic, I crossed it off twice, once on the notebook paper and then on the whiteboard. Let me not fail to mention that my editor had made up a nicely typed list of what needed still to be written, so actually I never even had to make the initial handwritten list in the first place!*

This is spending time on non-productive activity. It was particularly inappropriate because at that time I was way behind the writing schedule.

Motivating Yourself to Complete Work

It can help to have incentives to get things done. I am fond of a mini-cupcake-per-section-written approach. Competing with yourself can also help. For each task, set a goal of how much time it will take to complete. The excitement is in trying to beat the clock and still do a good job.

You can use a timer in a different way by setting the timer for a short amount of time, say 15 or 20 minutes. Promise yourself that you will only work that long. Usually that is doable. Then take a 10- to 15-minute break and do another 15- to 20- minute work session. As you repeat this you might find yourself just continuing to work.

Don't work for many hours at a stretch unless you are positive you can get the project done in one sitting. If you work a long time one day, you will not want to work on the project the next day and maybe even more days after that because you will have burned yourself out.

Meeting Other Work Challenges

The workplace requires more than getting projects done on time and to standard. You need to conform to the culture at large—the demands of meetings, the work environment (the office/desk/cubicle/workstation), and appropriate ways of communicating with colleagues and bosses.

Anticipate and Be Prepared

People with ADHD tend not to anticipate things, even if they have happened before. For example, you have a weekly staff meeting where you are always asked about the status of your projects. Even though this happens every week, you may not think to gather the information you need before the meeting starts unless you have been explicitly asked to do so.

Stay Vigilant!

In our journey to complete a long-term project we are continually coming upon patches of quicksand.

Once we manage to step across one, another patch of quicksand is waiting on the other side. Vigilance is required at all stages of the journey. We cannot let down our guard until the task or project is completely done. Before we get to completely done we encounter more quicksand, as we tend to stop before the project is fully done to the best of our ability within the allotted timeframe.

Practice anticipating what you will need to do to prepare for upcoming activities. One of the best ways to do this is to check on what you will need to complete, review what you are in the middle of, and go over what you have recently completed.

Don't rely on your memory alone. If you are going to be in a situation where someone will want to know the status of what you are working on, make a State of the Union list. This captures the status of all of your projects. Even if you don't end up needing it, it will help you get a sense of where you are with your projects and can help keep you on track.

Keep an Uncluttered Workspace

At work you are being judged by everything you do or don't do. People inside and outside your own organization are judging you, including by what your workstation looks like and how quickly you can find something.

People affected by ADHD often don't put things away, which leads to cluttered workstations. Since many people assume a cluttered space means a cluttered mind, anything we can do to appear in control of ourselves and our space is important.

Find a Home for What You Need

Be ruthless about what you actually need to get your work done and get rid of the rest. Then figure out a home for everything in your workstation.

Have Key Information Readily at Hand

Develop a simple system to access key information that you need to do your job. Keep in mind that if the system is too complicated you will not use it or keep it up to date. This system could be a binder with copies of templates and company guidelines or maybe a computer file where the tools of your trade are stored. (If you keep it on the computer, be sure to have a back up.) This system shouldn't take you a lot of time to put together. Don't get caught up in formatting and making it pretty. Put the information you need in your file and leave it at that.

The purpose of the file is to create an outline of your job and your responsibilities and is an easy reference point in case you forget or can't find something you need to do your job. It is also an important tool in case of emergencies. For example, if you are hospitalized, you can direct someone to this file to make sure key functions still get done.

If you have a poor memory for numbers and are often asked to provide them, develop a cheat sheet and keep it updated. Keep copies where you can access them. That way you will never be caught on the phone or with a client without an answer about such things as costs or program dates. You can also develop cheat sheets detailing procedures and contact information.

Interacting with Colleagues

When working with other people it is important to see yourself from their perspective. Consider making a list of questions to help you remember your usual blind spots when dealing with colleagues. Some of mine include:

- *Am I monopolizing the conversation?*
- *Am I being careful not to over share in a way that could be detrimental to me?*
- *Am I remembering that if I say it to one person, I'm really saying it to many?*
- *Am I being too blunt?*
- *Am I assuming I know more than this person?*
- *Am I listening for what I could learn from this person's experience?*

Write down your questions so that you can look at them and remind yourself that you are working towards becoming more aware of other people's perspectives. The more you work on this, the better you will get.

Managing Emotions

A lot of us with ADHD have difficulty managing our emotions at work. We feel things deeply, if sometimes fleetingly. Fortunately, we usually manage to move quickly away from the extreme emotion (we can give people whiplash with how quickly we go from one strong emotion to another). Unfortunately, while we are feeling the emotion we have a hard time hiding it and not acting on how we feel. This can cause us either to act rashly or to be judged by our peers and superiors as being ineffective at work because of our perceived lack of control.

The challenge in work situations is maintaining a calm exterior when inside you may want to cry, yell, laugh, or stew. If you feel like you are going to lose it, remove yourself from the situation as quickly as possible without causing waves. There are many ways to do this:

- *Simply say, "I will be right back." Don't explain further. Go to the restroom to collect yourself or if you have a private office, go in and relax. When you return, if you feel it is necessary, have something in your hand to act as though you left to get it.*

- *Be straight forward and say that you need a moment to think about what has been said before you continue the conversation. Or say that you believe a break would be helpful before continuing so that everyone can clear their heads. One of the best things you can do during a break is take a short walk, go outside, or preferably both.*

- *Write it down. In a meeting if I am feeling upset and I can't leave, I start writing down what I can do to solve the situation. I put down as many ideas as I can. This distracts me from my emotional response. I tear up easily, and this gets me actively moving toward a more neutral reaction. Also when you are writing you tend to look down, which hides your eyes. That can be helpful in not letting everyone in on how you are feeling. Be careful though not to duck your head too low, because that can send a negative message.*

At work it is important to manage your emotions and maintain control. If you encounter strong emotions, there are ways to manage the situation.

Getting Beyond Overwhelmed

Sometimes, even a lot of times, you will feel overwhelmed. One of the places this often happens is at work. It doesn't matter if you work for somebody else or you work for yourself, being overwhelmed can paralyze you. What can you do about it?

- **First, Get Organized!** *What are all the things you believe you need to do? Write them down. Write down everything that is in your head.*
- **Second, Be Critical**—*of your list, not yourself! Is everything on that list really necessary? Is there anything on it you can delegate, postpone, or just drop from the list because the return on the investment will be too small as compared to the time and effort it would take to do it?*
- **Third, Prioritize!** *Ask yourself what on that list is most critical and most time sensitive? What is the second most critical and time sensitive, and so forth. If you are not sure, ask someone for advice. Or, if you're stuck, just do the easiest and quickest tasks first. Success breeds momentum.*
- **Fourth, Dig In!** *Get started knocking out things on the list based on how you prioritized it. For each task, if you are struggling to get it done, start with the three smallest baby steps you can take and hopefully that will get you going. If that doesn't do it, do three more baby steps, etc.*
- **Fifth, Celebrate!** *Celebrate every win, no matter how small. Be your own cheerleader.*

These strategies will help you get unstuck and take on overwhelm at work. Don't let it defeat you! Realize that you can develop ways to take on the many challenges you face at work. You not only have techniques and approaches at hand, you also have the persistence and determination to pick yourself up when you fall down. You are not alone.

Forget Perfect

Consider feedback as information on actions, not a commentary on you as a person.

Don't put off work just because you don't know where to start.

Get to work, meetings, etc. on time.

Make a positive impression: keep your work area neat and uncluttered.

Set up simple systems for finding the information you need for your job.

Recognize that rules that apply to employees in your organization apply to you too.

Don't lose it at work. Keep your emotions in check or excuse yourself from a difficult situation.

Chapter Eleven

You Are Not Alone

My **hope is that this book** has given you ideas and actions you can take to help you live a happier life. However, actions alone only work in the presence of an attitude, an approach to life that I see in so many of the people I work with. Their lives are defined by resilience, persistence, and moving ahead in spite of difficulties.

Those of us with ADHD tend not to acknowledge or see these qualities in ourselves. But they are right there in front of us and within us.

ADHD may not be a gift, but you are. And you are not alone. *Everyone* has something, some kind of struggle in life, not just those of us with ADHD. My best advice is to forget perfect, choose to think and live in an anticipatory manner, and do things even if they don't feel "natural." What moves you forward in life is focusing on what you can do, not on what you can't. Don't get stuck thinking how hard something is. Yes, it may be, but you are more resourceful than you know. Don't worry so much about what other people are thinking. Keep your eye on what you want to achieve. You may just achieve it.

Think Future Life, Not Past Failures

Those of us with ADHD tend to focus on past failures rather than on future possibilities. Instead of looking backwards, think of your life as you want it to be.

We can take something precious from our past failures to bring into the future if we choose to do so. Our resiliency. When things go wrong, or not exactly as we planned, we keep going. Many people don't. That is a gift. Use it. Value it.

Focus on Success

You will encounter failures. Everyone does—even people without ADHD. Consider failure as part of the journey. The important thing is that when you do fail, you don't get stuck dwelling on the failure.

WRONG = *I have ADHD and so I fail at things*

Having ADHD means turning the equation upside down! Focus instead on what you have accomplished, no matter how small (or big) those accomplishments are.

RIGHT = *Despite ADHD I manage to achieve victories that make me stronger. The road may be a little tougher for me but I keep on going!*

Acknowledge that you are tough, relentless, and resilient.

The road may be a little tougher for me but I keep on going!

Life is not easy, but if you focus on "I can't," then you won't. If you focus on "despite...I do," an internal shift occurs. That shift includes acceptance that you need help for some things, acknowledgment that other things you can do yourself, and recognition that you can realize possibilities as yet unknown to you and to others. Finally, see that you are stronger for your experiences, not less than because of them.

See Yourself as More, Not Less

That positive view of life experiences also extends to how we present ourselves. Many of us with ADHD tend to be self-deprecators. We think that by being self-deprecating we are being modest, creating a simpatico vibe, like we are everyman or everywoman. But by being self-deprecating we are setting ourselves up as less than. Others begin to think of us as less than and then we begin to think of ourselves as less than, too.

Don't train people—or yourself—to think of you as less than you are. Train them to see your brilliance. We all are brilliant in our own unique way. Instead of putting yourself down privately or publicly, lift yourself up. Lifting yourself up in your own eyes will lift you up in the eyes of others.

Make Your Mark, Others Have

You have probably already heard of celebrities who have ADHD but here's a partial list of many influential people believed to have had or have ADHD.

Abraham Lincoln
Albert Einstein
Alexander Graham Bell
Andrew Carnegie
Bill Gates
David Neeleman
Dwight Eisenhower
Eleanor Roosevelt
Frank Lloyd Wright
George W. Bush
Gen. George Patton
Gen. William Westmoreland
George H. W. Bush
Henry Ford
James Carville
John F. Kennedy
Malcolm Forbes
Nelson Rockefeller
Richard Branson
Robert F. Kennedy
Ted Turner
Thomas Edison
Thomas Jefferson
Walt Disney
William Randolph Hearst
Woodrow Wilson

Those listed include political and military leaders, scientists, industrialists, inventors, and innovators. These people have made their mark both in spite of and because of ADHD. You can too.

Showing Up

Making your mark begins with participating in life and not letting anxiety about what will happen get the best of you.

When you have ADHD, you tend to avoid unpleasant situations and tasks because—and I know this sounds contradictory—you can think too far in advance, trying to figure out what will happen before it does.

...This will lead to that, which will lead to that, which will lead to that...

Somewhere in that string may be something you aren't sure you know how to do or want to do. So why start this domino effect? Why indulge in this kind of anxious future thinking?

In this case only, *don't* think ahead. Just show up. Simply be present and commit to staying present. Sometimes things won't go well, but if you keep showing up you will find that most of the time they do. Even more important is that the more you show up in life, the easier life becomes. You'll get more accomplished, and you'll be there for other people more often.

Keep showing up and being present in your life. Amazing things will happen.

The Best You Can Do Is The Best You Can Do

No matter how far you move forward, you still are who you were when you started your journey. I am an ADHD coach and I have progressed in my life since I found out about my ADHD in my 30s. Although I have aggressively sought treatment, I am still the same person. I have made many steps forward but every once in awhile I fall way back.

You will get off track because of your ADHD. It's going to happen. Just move on, move ahead. Maybe even laugh at your missteps once in awhile. You're not perfect. Nobody is.

> *Congratulations to me! Despite ADHD, I had a good day and really accomplished a lot. Set out in morning very determined to focus on what I needed to get done. Took a few short breaks. Didn't get as far as I had hoped but so often*

I can be unrealistic as to what I can accomplish in a day. Dwelling in the energy of what I did do is a better place for me to be. It helps me approach tomorrow with a positive attitude.

There Is No "Right Way"

Sometimes when you have ADHD you think you are doing things the "right way" and this right way seems to be working. You've got your list of things you have planned to get done and you're on schedule, going right through it. Then you let go, just for a minute or something gets you off course and things start to fall apart. The kind of rigidity born of this right way/wrong way thinking can quickly cause a downward spiral.

My day is tightly packed with everything I want to accomplish. I have allotted 20 minutes for breakfast and washing dishes, 5 minutes for a phone call to my doctor's office, 5 minutes to leave the house, and 30 minutes to get to the cleaners—and this is just from 8 am to 9 am. But when I call the doctor, they put me on hold. I am annoyed and stressed because it's now 10 minutes on the phone and I still don't have the information I was calling about. I'm starting to melt down because I feel everything I planned falling to pieces around me. I had it all mapped out but now I'm already behind in my day.

I have some clients who are hyperorganized and hypervigilant because they are so afraid their ADHD will cause them to make a mistake. Their rigidity can be their downfall because once a little crack occurs in the armor, it shatters.

Being more flexible allows for bends and flows and makes you able to absorb the occasional blow or mistake and still keep moving forward. When I was on the phone I could have decided to hang up and call back later, or simply realize I wasn't going to make it to the dry cleaners today.

Leave some space in life for the mistakes and blows—some small, others bigger. These are inevitable. Just remember you can absorb them and move onward.

Becoming Future Oriented

Those of us with ADHD live mostly in the moment. Remember that Dr. Ned Hallowell, who co-wrote two of the best-known books about ADHD, put it like this, "For people affected by ADHD, there is now and not now."

While living in the present you may also worry that catastrophe is just around the corner if anything goes wrong. This may be because you have only enough money to meet your basic needs and nothing else. Emergencies can happen. Think of the future and give yourself a cushion, whether it's financial, personal, or professional. By always working towards building your future, you can develop confidence that you can deal with most unexpected situations.

If the Plane is Going Down, I Want You Sitting Next to Me

When we talk about ADHD, we talk about the deficits. What we can't do. How we fail. We talk about the frustration we feel and the frustration others feel with ourselves and our repeated mistakes, like being late. No matter how hard we try or how often we promise to do better, we often slip up again.

But if a plane were going down, we would kick ass. There are exceptions, but most of the people I have met with ADHD are great in emergencies. We do well under pressure because it stimulates us. It's important to remind ourselves of what we do well, recognize it, and use it as a guide.

Don't feel down about all the little things that you have trouble doing. Remember, when it comes to the big stuff in life, the truly important stuff, anyone in their right mind would want you by their side.

There is a hero inside you even if you are never called to action, so stand tall!

Before the Curtain Falls

In closing there are three things I want to leave you with:

- ***Resist Resistance***
- ***Remind Yourself That There Is No Secret Rule Book***
- ***Get Back on the Train***

Resist Resistance

Little has been written about resistance in this book, but it is a big issue for people affected by ADHD. We don't like being told what to do and therefore we often become resistant to doing whatever we have been told to do.

> *I was about to make a call to my doctor's office when my mom called and said, "Did you call the doctor yet?" Shoot, I thought, now I won't be calling him today. I knew it was ridiculous but for some reason her call "nagging me" shut me down. My "resistance shackles" came up and I knew I would not make the call that day, even though it would be detrimental to myself not to.*

All I can tell you about resistance is try to resist it. Seriously. When you feel it coming on, question it. Is it in your best interest to resist? Are you resisting doing something you were already going to do just because someone also told you to do it? Are you being plain stubborn? Is there another way you can find an entry point to the situation that cools it down?

When we feel resistance, all we are doing is resisting helping ourselves.

The Secret Rulebook

I have discovered that many people affected by ADHD believe that there is some secret rulebook that everyone else has but them. This is a rulebook either that they alone didn't get or people affected by ADHD didn't get.

Here is the truth:

There is no secret rulebook.

Everyone, whether they are affected by ADHD or not, is making it up as they go along. Life is one grand improvisation with all of us learning on the job. No one is exempt from the uncertainty inherent in this experiment.

Get Back on The Train

There is an important skill you need to learn when you have ADHD and that is *get back on the train quickly*.

When we are trying to change our behaviors, accomplish new things, or make mental shifts, we often fall off the train in the process. Instead of getting back up, dusting ourselves off, and recommitting by getting right back on the train, we waste time self-flagellating as the train moves on. Then we have to either run and catch up with it or simply decide to quit.

As I explain it to my clients, most of whom are located in the Washington D.C. area, you get on the train at Union Station (in Washington, D.C.), travel through Maryland, and then fall off the train in Delaware. Now you have a choice. You can get back on the train in Philadelphia, the next major stop, or you can spend your energy and time bemoaning the fact that you fell off the train, getting mad at yourself about it, and thinking negative, judgmental thoughts about yourself.

Granted, not falling off the train in the first place would be best, but all growth, change, and forward movement comes with some pain. It is how you handle that pain that matters. Do you want to intensify it and delay your life's journey by judging yourself, or do you simply dust yourself off and jump back on the train and keep on keeping on? I advocate for the latter.

Besides, that perfect world you think exists? It's kind of boring. Maybe in that world you'd never fall off the train in the first place, but what kind of a story would that make? I think your story, your journey, is likely to be more interesting and adventurous when you fall, get up, and keep on moving. Forget perfect. In the end, letting go of perfection will give you a much more rewarding and (ironically) easier life.

Forget Perfect

Train others to see your brilliance.

You have unbelievable resilience. You do not let failure defeat you.

If you're more flexible, less rigid, you can absorb the occasional letdown more easily.

Show up. Be present in your life.

Give yourself a cushion for the future.

Appendix A: Basic Treatment for ADHD

Before you seek treatment for ADHD it is important to get a diagnosis from a psychiatrist because they can treat ADHD with medication, which works for 70% of those who try it. Medication for most then will be part of a multi-modal treatment plan.

Multi-Modal Treatment

Once you get a diagnosis, a multi-modal treatment plan is most effective for those diagnosed with ADHD. Your plan can include your doctor to monitor your treatment plan, a coach if you feel you need support to move forward or to work on behavioral issues, a therapist like a psychologist if you have co-morbidities (other related difficulties such as depression, anxiety, OCD, conduct disorder), which are common for people affected by ADHD or if you feel there are issues/feelings related to ADHD that you need to talk about.

Your treatment plan should also include exercise, which stimulates important chemicals in your brain. You also need good nutrition and adequate sleep. Sleep may be difficult as sleeping issues often occur when you are affected by ADHD. You must also be free of unhealthy addictions.

I am not medically trained, but what I present here is a framework that has worked for me and many of my clients. Please note that the reader should not stop any treatments they are currently receiving for ADHD or start any new treatments for ADHD without first checking with their doctor.

I think of the multi-modal treatment plan for people affected by ADHD as my Hand Plan. It includes five things, listed in no particular order:

- *Psychiatrist (for prescriptions, therapy, if they do it)*
- *Therapist, social worker, and/or coach*
- *Medication (if it works for you)*
- *Exercise plan (check with your doctor first)*
- *Good sleep*

You don't have to limit yourself to five modalities and they don't have to be these, but it is a good start. The last modality listed, good sleep, is often a difficulty for people affected by ADHD and poor sleep can make symptoms of ADHD worse. If you don't have this problem, I suggest substituting good nutrition for good sleep. Good nutrition is generally important, but if you are starting out with a plan for treating ADHD, only add one thing at a time.

Psychiatrist

Keeping with the metaphor of the hand, the first finger I recommend is seeing a psychiatrist rather than a general practitioner to diagnose ADHD and prescribe medication. Psychiatrists are medical doctors who typically know more than general practitioners (GPs) about the various medications that work with ADHD. Also, many GPs will shy away from prescribing stimulants, even though these have a higher success rate for treating ADHD symptoms than other non-stimulant medications developed specifically for ADHD. Some psychiatrists do talk therapy and some don't. If your psychiatrist does not and you have one of the common co-morbidities associated with ADHD you should be treated by a specialist.The co-morbidities include but are not limited to depression, anxiety, substance abuse and oppositional disorders.

Psychologist, Social Worker, and/or Coach

The next finger of the hand plan is getting someone who can help you take actions in your life that can support you. A psychologist can help you with emotional issues and provide behavioral therapy. A social worker can help you find services and people to help you. Social workers have some training in mental health but not as much as psychologists.

A coach helps you take actions to move your life forward. Many people who see a psychiatrist or psychologist also see a coach. Unlike the practitioners discussed above, there is no special training or education that's required before someone can call themselves a coach. For this reason, when engaging a coach it is best to find a coach trained in ADHD coaching and certified by the International Coaches Federation (ICF). (For more information on what coaching is and how to find good ADHD coaches, see Appendix D).

Medication

The third finger represents medication which has been very successful in helping people manage their ADHD symptoms. The greatest success has been found with stimulants. For those who fear addiction to stimulants, some studies have shown that those who take stimulants are less likely to have addiction problems than those who do not take medication for ADHD. It is thought that those not taking medication are self-medicating with drugs or alcohol.

Medication does not cure ADHD. Just as cold and allergy medicine treats the symptoms of the cold or allergy, it does not cure the allergies or cold. The same is true with ADHD. Stimulants help with some of the difficulties that ADHD causes but when the stimulant wears off the symptoms return. Whether you take 1 day of stimulant pills or 300 days, you will still have the symptoms of ADHD if you stop taking the stimulant.

I advocate for the use of medication because it has made a profound difference in my own ability to initiate tasks, complete tasks, and work on long-term projects. I could never have written a book prior to getting medication treatment for my

ADHD because I couldn't focus. It has also made a difference in my compulsive talking. I am still a verbal person, but my talking is no longer out of control. Moreover, I work for myself, which involves a lot of self-motivation, which I don't think I would have had prior to my ADHD treatment. Someone else may not get the same benefits, but medication has definitely changed my life for the better.

Exercise

The second to the last finger of the hand plan is exercise. It is hard to exercise regularly, but it is important to do so. With exercise your body releases chemicals that help you focus. Exercise is also important because it calms those of us who are hyperactive. It is like getting free medicine, and you don't want to waste that!

Any kind of activity will do as long as some portion of it is aerobic, that is, your heart rate is elevated for portions of the activity. You don't need equipment or a gym membership. Jumping jacks or walking at a brisk pace are free. This is part of the treatment plan that is a no-brainer!

When you exercise you grow new neurons, which helps with some executive functions. Exercise also reduces the risk of diabetes and obesity--not things to dismiss. John Ratey, a Harvard Medical School neuropsychiatrist who wrote *Spark: The Revolutionary Science of Exercise and the Brain*, devotes a chapter in his book to ADHD. "Ratey describes BDNF[11] as 'Miracle-Gro for the brain' because it creates an environment where neurons can flourish and promotes the formation of new connections between cells."[12]

Some time ago it was believed that if you did crossword puzzles and brain teasers as you got older it would help you stay sharp. There is actually not a lot of evidence supporting this. "In contrast, new exercise regimes tend to accelerate processing speed and improve attention and memory in all kinds of activities,"[13] according to Arthur Kramer, a cognitive psychologist at the Beckman Institute for Advanced Science and Technology at the University of Illinois.

11. BDNF - Brain-derived neurotrophic factor
12. Washington Post 12/10/13 E5
13. ibid

If you are affected by ADHD the likelihood of dementia is slightly higher than it is for the average bear. There are no guarantees that you can prevent this from happening, but there is something simple that you can do to reduce the risk of dementia, improve your cognitive abilities, and enhance your overall sense of well-being.

Good Sleep

It has become clear that sleep is key for people affected by ADHD. Some experts are even starting to believe that some of the people diagnosed with ADHD might instead have ADHD symptoms because of chronic lack of sleep. The majority of my clients have difficulty getting enough sleep so good sleep hygiene is important.

With the Hand Plan, the five modalities work together. One final recommendation I don't include on the hand because it is so self-evident and applies to everyone, ADHD or not: Don't smoke or stop smoking if you are a smoker.

No Smoking!

Many people affected by ADHD self-medicate through alcohol, drugs, and smoking. I put smoking in the same group as drugs because nicotine is an addictive substance. While it may calm you temporarily, it will kill you in the end. Fifty percent of ADHD people smoke at some point, and it hurts them in more than the obvious ways. It often defines who becomes and stays their friends, whether they get a job (employers can smell it on them), or get picked for an athletic team.

It is simple: if you don't smoke, don't start. If you do smoke, get help now. The sooner, the better. The longer you smoke, the harder it will be to quit. Not only can you die of lung cancer, but it can cause other illnesses. I have seen the damage smoking can do. It compromises your body, especially your respiratory system. If your lungs are damaged by smoking, you are more likely to develop complications that can lead to death. There is some good news. Even if you have smoked for awhile, quitting will add years to your life.

Appendix B: ADHD and Related Organizations

ADHD Coaches Organization (ACO)
www.adhdcoaches.org
Membership organization for ADHD coaches, which includes a directory of ADHD coaches.

Attention Deficit Disorder Association (ADDA)
www.add.org
Membership organization for adults with ADHD. Also has a coach directory.

Children and Adults with Attention Deficit (CHADD)
www.chadd.org
Membership organization for children, adults, and parents of people with ADHD; also has the National Resource Center (NRC) on ADHD, which is a repository of information on ADHD. Has a coach directory.

National Resource Center on ADHD (NRC)
www.Help4adhd.org

National Alliance on Mental Illness (NAMI)
www.nami.org
Advocacy and support regarding mental illness; has information regarding ADHD.

ADHD AWARENESS
www.adhdawarenessmonth.org
Collaborative effort to bring awareness about ADHD during ADHD awareness month (February).

International Coach Federation (ICF)
www.coachfederation.org
Foremost certifying organization for coaches; has listing of certified coaches.

National Institute of Mental Health (NIMH)

nimh.nih.gov

Scientific organization dedicated to the understanding, treatment, and prevention of mental disorders.

American Psychological Association (APA)

www.apa.org/topics/adhd/index.aspx

Association of psychologists and publishing house for psychological topics, including ADHD.

Appendix C: Recommended Books By Topic

This list highlights books that can give you good basic knowledge of subjects related to ADHD. It is by no means exhaustive.

As you read these books and find others, remember that just as with my book, many ADHD books are written from personal points of view. This means that you'll likely find differing opinions and contradictory ideas. Use the books you find on ADHD as a guide, not as a replacement for seeking treatment from a medical doctor or psychologist.

General ADHD

Brown, Thomas E. *Attention Deficit Disorder: The Unfocused Mind in Children and Adults.* New Haven: Yale University Press, 2005.

Hallowell, Edward M. and John J. Ratey. *Delivered from Distraction: Getting the Most Out of Life with Attention Deficit Disorder*. New York: Ballantine Books, 2006.

Hallowell, Edward M. and John J. Ratey. *Driven to Distraction: Recognizing and Coping with Attention Deficit Disorder from Childhood through Adulthood.* Rev. Ed. New York: Anchor Books, 2011.

Kelly, Kate and Peggy Ramundo. *You Mean I'm Not Lazy, Stupid or Crazy: The Classic Self-Help Book for Adults with Attention Deficit Disorder.* Rev. Ed. New York: Scribner, 2006.

Executive Functions

Barkley, Russell A. *Executive Functions.* New York: Guilford Press. 2012.

Brown, Thomas E. *A New Understanding of ADHD in Children and Adults: Executive Function Impairments.* New York: Routledge, 2013.

Moraine, Paula. *Helping Students Take Control of Everyday Executive Functions.* Philadelphia: Jessica Kingsley, 2012.

Adults

Barkley, Russell A. *Taking Charge of Adult ADHD.* New York: Guilford Press, 2010.

Leverini, Abigail and Frances Prevatt. *Succeeding with Adult ADHD: Daily Strategies to Help You Achieve Your Goals and Manage Your Life.* Washington D.C.: American Psychological Association, 2012.

Murphy, Kevin R. *Out of the Fog: Treatment Options and Coping Strategies for Adult Attention Deficit Disorder.* New York: Hyperion. 1995.

Tuckman, Ari. *More Attention, Less Deficit: Success Strategies for Adults with ADHD.* Plantation: Specialty Press, 2009.

Zylowska, Lidia. *The Mindfulness Prescription for Adult ADHD.* Boston: Trumpeter Books. 2012.

Women

Matlen, Terry. *The Queen of Distraction: How Women with ADHD Can Conquer Chaos, Find Focus, and Get More Done.* Oakland: New Harbinger Publications, 2014.

Solden, Sari. *Women with Attention Deficit Disorder: Embrace Your Differences and Transform Your Life.* Rev. and exp. ed. Nevada City, CA: Underwood Books, 2005.

Youth

Spodak, Ruth and Kenneth Stefano. *Take Control of ADHD.* Waco, TX: Prufrock Press. 2011.

For Parents with ADHD Children

Barkley, Russell A. *Taking Charge of ADHD: The Complete, Authoritative Guide for Parents.* New York: Guilford Press, 2013.

Brown, Thomas E. *Smart but Stuck: Emotions in Teens and Adults with ADHD.* San Francisco: Jossey-Bass, 2014.

Cooper-Kahn and Laurie Dietzel. *Late, Lost, and Unprepared: A Parents' Guide to Helping Children with Executive Functioning.* Bethesda: Woodbine House, 2008.

Dawson, Peg and Richard Guare. *Smart but Scattered.* New York: Guilford Press, 2009.

Ford, Anne and John-Richard Thompson. *On Their Own*. New York: Newmarket Press. 2007.

Heininger, Janet E. and Sharon K. Weiss. *From Chaos to Calm*. New York: Penguin Group. 2001.

Science of ADHD

Barkley, Russell, Kevin R. Murphy and Mariellen Fischer. *ADHD in Adults: What the Science Says*. New York: Guilford Press, 2008.

Finance

Sarkis, Stephanic Moulton and Karl Klein. *ADD and Your Money*. Oakland: New Harbinger Publications, 2009.

Couples

Maucieri, Larry and Jon Carlson, Eds. *The Distracted Couple: The Impact of ADHD on Adult Relationships*. Bethel, CT: Crown House Publishing, 2014.

Orlov, Melissa. *The ADHD Effect on Marriage*. Plantation, FL: Specialty Press, 2010.

Orlov, Melissa and Nancie Kohlenberger. *The Couple's Guide to Thriving with ADHD*. Plantation, FL: Specialty Press, 2014.

Pera, Gina. *Is It You, Me, or Adult A.D.D.?* San Francisco: 1201 Alarm Press, 2008.

Social Issues

Novotni, Michele. *What Does Everybody Else Know That I Don't?* Plantation, FL: Specialty Press. 2008.

Organizing

Kolberg, Judith and Kathleen Nadeau. *ADD-Friendly Ways to Organize Your Life*. New York: Brunner-Routledge. 2002.

Pinsky, Susan C. *Organizing Solutions for People with ADHD*. Beverly: Fair Winds Press, 2012.

Ratey, Nancy. *The Disorganized Mind: Coaching Your ADHD Brain to Take Control of Your Time, Tasks & Talents*. New York: St. Martin's Griffin, 2008.

Miscellaneous ADHD

Richardson, Wendy. *When Too Much Isn't Enough*. Colorado Springs: NavPress, 2005.

The following books do not specifically address ADHD but are helpful for those with ADHD and relate to what is covered in this book.

Couples

Hallowell, Edward, Sue Hallowell and Melissa Orlov. *Married to Distraction: Restoring Intimacy and Strengthening Your Marriage in an Age of Interruption*. New York: Ballantine Books, 2010.

Parker-Pope, Tara. *For Better: How the Surprising Science of Happy Couples Can Help Your Marriage Succeed*. New York: Penguin Group, 2010.

Emotional/Social Issues

Moran, Victoria. *Shelter for the Spirit*. New York: HarperCollins, 1997.

Productivity

Covey, Stephen R. *First Things First: To Live, to Love, to Learn, to Leave a Legacy.* New York: Simon & Schuster, 1995.

Covey, Stephen R. *The Seven Habits of Highly Effective People: Powerful Lessons on Personal Change.* New York: Simon & Schuster, 1989.

Career Issues

Eikleberry, Carol. *The Career Guide for Creative and Unconventional People.* Berkeley: Ten Speed Press. 1999.

Feldman, Wilma R. *Finding a Career That Works For You.* Plantationm FL: Specialty Press, 2006.

Sher, Barbara. *I Could Do Anything: If I Only Knew What It Was.* New York: Dell, 1994.

Appendix D: ADHD Coaching

FAQs

This section answers questions about ADHD coaching.

What can ADHD coaching do for you?

Having ADHD can be hard. All your life you have been told that you are lazy, impulsive, unfocused, forgetful, or unmotivated. You may have even begun to feel you aren't very smart. Your life may feel chaotic and unstructured.

An ADHD coach will help you create more structure in your life and will help you conquer some of the roadblocks you encounter because of ADHD. A coach expert in ADHD will understand the issues that confront you daily and will be trained to coach to those issues.

One caveat: coaching, as in most things, only works if the person is all in. This is true with life. Your life only works both professionally and personally if you are all in, showing up, and being present.

How is coaching defined?

Coaching is an interdevelopmental relationship between client and coach. It is a partnership of equals. The coach is expert on coaching and the client is expert on him or herself. It is assumed that the client is whole, competent, creative, and intelligent. Unlike therapy, consulting, or mentorship, the client is not in a one down position from the expert therapist, consultant, or mentor. Again, the client is assumed to have no pathology.

Yet ADHD is a pathology, just like diabetes is a pathology. So some coaches do not believe in ADHD coaching because the ADHD client is not considered "whole" and is counted out due to their ADHD and possible ancillary issues.

An ADHD coach does not have this view and should be expert in ADHD and working with ADHD clients.

Why hire an ADHD coach?

ADHD coaching starts from where you are in your life and looks to the goals you wish to achieve in life: long-term, medium-term, or even short-term.

If you are not sure of your goals, you can hire an ADHD coach to help you figure out what they are. ADHD coaching supports you in what you wish to do. You set the agenda. The coach helps you pursue that agenda.

You might ask how does an ADHD coach do that?

The coach helps you change habits, develop systems, work on how you make choices, get unstuck when you are stuck, simplify when complexities get in the way of life, and if you wish, be more accountable. These are just some of the things an ADHD coach can help you with.

What is ADHD coaching?

ADHD coaching helps the ADHD client develop a more structured and goal-oriented life. The coach, who specializes in ADHD, can help the client work on executive function skills, learn about ADHD, and manage life better.

How often does the coaching happen?

Usually ADHD coaching happens in one session a week, especially in the beginning. Coaching can also happen every other week or once a month. The frequency of the coaching is really up to you and your coach.

How long does a coaching session last?

A coaching session lasts 30 to 60 minutes, depending on the coach and the client.

What is an intake session?

With many ADHD coaches, after you sign up you begin your sessions. Some coaches, like myself, schedule a longer initial "intake session." These sessions range from 90 minutes to 2 hours. They often include an introduction to ADHD coaching, completion of necessary paperwork, assessments the coach might want to administer, and determination of your goals for being coached. These sessions jumpstart the coach-client relationship and allow coach and client to get to work immediately in the regular sessions.

Where does the coaching take place?

The coaching takes place in person, over the phone, Skype, and email. This depends on how the coach works and what the client wants.

What role does ADHD coaching play in a family or couple?

An ADHD coach takes responsibility out of the hands of the spouse or parents to constantly monitor the ADHD behavior so that they can just be a spouse or a parent and not have to play the dual roles of loved one and "enforcer/monitor." That becomes a negative experience for both the ADHD member of the family and the parent or spouse. The coach allows everyone to play their natural roles and maintain positive relationships rather than relationships filled with nagging, conflict, and disappointment.

Hiring an ADHD Coach

You're ready for ADHD coaching, but don't know how or whom to hire? First, strike while the iron is hot. Don't put it off. When you know you are ready, start looking immediately before the notion becomes less immediate.

Get a Personal Recommendation, If Available

A good way to hire an ADHD coach is through a personal recommendation from a doctor, therapist, social worker, fellow person affected by ADHD or someone else who knows you. But often that is not possible. The following are the steps to take to find ADHD coaches.

Selecting and Vetting from Listings of Coaches

You can find websites that list ADHD coaches. The most well-known listings are provided below. You'll find ADHD coaches usually listed under "resources" or "support."

www.adhdcoaches.org

The ADHD Coaches Organization (ACO) is a professional organization for ADHD coaches. (I think this is the best site because to be a professional member you must have a prescribed minimal level of training; full disclosure, I am on their board of directors.) The downside of the ACO listing is that it is not large.

www.chadd.org

CHADD (Children and Adults with Attention Deficit Disorder) is the largest ADHD organization and also has a coach listing. There are no criteria to be listed. As with all the listing sites, coaches pay to be listed.

www.add.org

ADDA (Attention Deficit Disorder Association) is an organization specifically devoted to adults with ADHD. I have noticed recently that they are expanding to reach out to the college student population.

www.additudemag.com

Additude is a quarterly print magazine (at the time of this writing) with a digital weekly magazine. Their website has a resource directory listing coaches. Coaches can pay for highlighted listings, which means they are not necessarily better than the other coaches listed.

How to Vet a Coach

Selecting a coach is an important decision. You need to spend time getting information, talking to prospective coaches, and taking into consideration their expertise and fit for working with you.

This is how to start:

- *Search the listings for the right type of coach for you. If you are interested in seeing a coach in person, rather than by phone or Skype, your first criterion likely will be location. If you prefer the phone, Skype, or there is not a coach in your immediate area, then the first criterion could be what the coach specializes in. (Some coaches may only work over the phone or Skype.)*
- *Review the listings and pick at least 3 coaches.*
- *Go to the coaches' websites to learn more about them. Look at the information rather than just the design of the website.*
- *Talk with a minimum of three coaches to get a sense of them and whether you can work with and trust them. (Each site will either have a contact link, phone number, or both.)*
- *Take notes about each coach you research and talk to so you can make an informed decision.*

The following is the information you want to find out from their website and during your conversations with them.

Who They Work With

- *What populations do they have experience ADHD coaching? Adults, adolescents, college students, couples, parents, etc.*
- *Do they have specific training with said populations?*

Training and Education

- *What is their coach training?*
- *What is their ADHD coach training?*
- *Do they continue their ADHD coaching education?*

Coaching Philosophy

- *What is their philosophy about ADHD?*
- *What is their philosophy about ADHD coaching?*

Experience and Programs

- *How long have they been ADHD coaching?*
- *Aside from one on one ADHD coaching, do they have other programs?*
- *If it matters to you, ask how they got involved with ADHD coaching, i.e. have ADHD themselves, parent of someone affected by ADHD, retired teacher, etc.*
- *Are they a member of any professional organizations such as the International Coaches Federation (the ICF)? Any ADHD specific organization? This means they have agreed to certain ethical standards and likely have an interest in professional development.*

Working with Clients

- *Are they immediately available for new clients?*
- *What are the days and hours they see clients?*
- *What are the costs for one on one coaching? Do they charge per session or do they have packages such as three months or 6 sessions?*
- *What comes with sessions or packages of sessions such as unlimited emails between sessions?*
- *What methods of payment do they take?*
- *When does the client pay?*
- *What are their policies for cancellations or re-scheduling?*
- *How long are the actual sessions?*

If you are considering a coach you would see in person, ask about transportation. Is public transportation near them, or is parking available where they are located? And also ask about issues of accessibility if you have any issues that impede your ability to see them.

Finally, do you feel like you connected with the coach while talking with them? It is important that the two of you are able to build a rapport on which to develop a relationship.

Hopefully this will be life changing so it is important that you do due diligence before making a decision.

Appendix E: Apps That Support People Diagnosed with ADHD

This list of apps is provided to help you find useful tools, systems, and support for what you are trying to accomplish. Since apps are frequently updated and new ones are released, go to www.abigailwurf.com/apps for an update to the apps listing.

I recommend that you download an app only after you have fully explored it, including reading reviews of it. Also, don't try to adopt too many of them. They can clutter up your devices and lead to storing similar information in many different locations. You also may find that you don't use them.

Note that many of these apps are free. Others require either making a one-time payment or paying for a subscription.

ADHD-Specific

Alarm Clock 4 (various alarms)
Concentrate (distraction elimination)
Elevate (brain training)
Eternity Time (time logging)
Focus Booster (Pomodoro timer)
Google Now (information management)
Morning (support for routines)
My Minutes (time tracking)
SelfControl (prevents website browsing distraction)
Sleep Cycle (identifies sleep cycles and wakes you up)
Forest: Stay Focused, Be Present (helps improve focus)
Time Tracker (time audit)
Top of the Morning (preparation for the day to come)

Communication

Agenda Calendar 4 (calendar with communication capacity)
Away Find (notifies you of important messages)
Box (share documents)
Dragon Dictation (voice recognition)
Dropbox (share documents)
Google Hangouts (individual and group or audio video calls)
Humin (your digital butler)
LogMeIn (remote desktop)
Skype (video and voice calls)
Slack (team communications)
Speek (conference call service with notes, screen sharing, and file sharing)
Universal Password Manager (manage passwords)

Financial Management

Acorns (investment)
Bill Organizer (manage and track bills)
BillGuard (money tracker)
EEBA- Easy Envelope Budget Aid (budgeting, envelope system)
Expensify (manage money, scan receipts)
Freshbooks (cloud accounting)
Grocery Pal (sales and coupons for selected stores)
Home Budget (home finances)
iXpenseIt (record expenses)
Learn Vest (financial planning)
Manilla (financial organizer)
Mint (budget management)
Mobile Banking Apps (check with your bank to see if available)
PayPal Mobility App (payment system)
Pocket Expense (track personal finances)
Quickbooks (accounting software)
Soulver (calculator)
Venmo (social payment system)
YNAB- You Need A Budget (budget helper)

Fitness-Related

Calorie Count (tracks exercise, also the consumption of food and water)
MyFitnessPal (count calories and track exercise)
RuntasticPro (track activity)
Steps (pedometer)

Focus-Supporting

Attention Exercise (focus exercises that use doodling to improve memory)
Concentrate (distraction elimination)
Elevate (brain training)
Focus Booster (Pomodoro time tracker)
Focus@Will (neuroscience and music to boost productivity)
Koi Pond (calming activity)
MyMinutes (time tracking)
Stay Focused (limits time on websites)
TrackTime (attention audit)

Home Management

BigOven (recipe organizer)
BrightNest (home organization, cleaning)
Chore Checklist (chore manager)
Cleaning Checklist (a cleaning checklist)
Cozi Family Organizer (sharing calendar and tasks)
EpicWin (gamification of chore management and completion)
Grocery Gadget (shopping list)
Grocery iQ (grocery lists)
HomeRoutines (schedules, lists, timer, "encourager")
Mealboard (recipe manager)
MotivatedMoms (chore planning)
My Things (productivity and file management)
PackingPro (planning for travel)
Simply Us (organize life together)
Savr (finds grocery deals)
TaskRabbit (people run errands and do home tasks for you)
UnfilthYourHabitat (motivation for cleaning home)

Information Management

1Password (password manager)
Awesome Note (+ToDo/task management)
Bento (organize contacts, events, projects & to-do lists)
Captio (email yourself fast)
Cloze (collects social media)
Dashlane (password)
Digg (news)
Drafts (note-taking apps)
Dropbox (share, access and store files)
Droplr (quick sharing of documents, photos etc.)
Evernote (note-taking, images, audio notes, organize by tags)
Feedly (news)
Flipboard (news)
GoodReader (PDF reader and editing tool)
GoogleDrive (access files)
Instapaper (strips ads)
iQue (tracks information)
LastPass (password manager)
Mention (like Google alerts, media monitoring)
Mindjet (mindmapping app that allows you to easily move between different sub topics and back again)
MindNode (mindmapping with cross-referencing to all maps; capability to publish them with MyMindNode service)
Momento (daily journal, take pictures, pulls feeds from social media)
OneDrive (remote access to files and photos)
OneNote (note-taking, lists, photo information that is searchable)
Pocket (save and share articles)
RE.minder (reminder with notes ability)
Reeder (news)

TextExpander (custom keyboard shortcuts to speed typing)
Threadnote (short note taking)
Trello (organizer)
Universal Password Manager (saves passwords)
Vesper (note-taking with tagging)

Logistical

1Password (password management)
Checkmark (to-do and task lists)
ConverterPlus (currencies, units and calculators)
GateGuru (travel)
Google Now (information management)
Hightail (move large files, email)
Hipmunk (travel)
Hotwire (car rentals)
KayakPro (travel)
LogMeIn (remote access and desktop)
MenuPages (restaurant menus)
Morning (support for routines)
OpenTable (make restaurant reservations)
Redlaser (shop)
Swiftkey (keyboard)
TripCase (trip planning and alerts)
TripIt (trip planner)
Yelp (reviews of local businesses)

Organizational

2Do (captures ideas, creates to-do lists)
Any.do (organizational and task management app with many other capabilities)
Bento (organizes contacts, events, projects and to-do lists)
Clear (tasks, reminders, and to-do lists)
Evernote (notes, research, expenses)
Mindnode (mindmapping and planning)
OneNote (note-taking)
Remember the Milk (tracks lists and tasks)
Trello (organizes tasks, projects, lists, can be shared)

Productivity

AwayFind (notifies you of important messages)
Checkmark (to-do and task list)
Do (run productive meetings)
Dragon Dictation (dictation: speaking is often quicker than typing)
Droplr (shares images, documents, files, and links)
EasilyDo (personal assistant)
Focus@Will (neuroscience and music to boost productivity)
Freckle (time tracking)
Goal Streaks (goals and habit tracker)
GoodReader (PDF reader and editing tool)
Google Drive (cloud storage and file backup)
HomeRoutines (schedules, lists, timer, "encourager" for repeats)
Ifttt (if this, then that)
Launchy (app launcher)
LogMeIn (remote access)
Mailbox (manages emails)
OmniFocus (task management and calendar)

Producteev (task management for teams)
SignNow (sign docs)
SugarSync (sync files)
TextExpander (typing shortcut)
Things (task management)

Project Management

Asana (collective communication)
Basecamp (multi platform team project management)
Fanurio (time tracking for freelancers)
Flow (collective communication)
Freckle (time tracking)
Podio (project management)
Tempo (calendar)
Todoist (to-do and task list)
Toodledo (productivity)
Trello (organizes tasks, projects, lists, can be shared)

Task Management

2Do (capable of color coding, reminders, links to contacts)
Any.do (task management)
Asana (team productivity)
Bloom (productivity)
Clear (tasks, reminders, to-do lists)
Do (run productive meetings)
Due (task management with alarm reminders)
Errands (categorizes tasks and allows you to set due dates and alarms)

Flow (team task management)
iPhone (sync alerts across your iPhone, iPad, and Mac to be reminded of to-do items wherever you are)
MyLifeOrganized (task manager)
Nirvana (productivity)
Orchestra To-do (shared to-do lists)
Priorities (task management)
Re.minder (reminder with notes ability)
Remember the Milk (tracks lists and tasks)
Routinely! (reminds you of daily routines and tracks success)
Tasks (task management)
TeuxDeux (to-do app)
Timeful (with calendar)
Todoist (to-do and task list)
Toodledo (productivity)
Trello (organizer)
Wunderlist (ability to share lists, reminders, attach photos and files to to-do lists)
Zendone (task manager)

Time Management

30/30 (task manager app with sequential countdown timers, helps you learn how long tasks take)
Agenda Calendar 4 (calendar)
Alarmdroid (alarm app with additional features)
ATracker (daily task and time tracking)
Calvetica Calendar (fast calendaring)
Clear (tasks, reminders, and to-do lists)
Dragon Dictation (dictate: speaking is often quicker than typing)
Eternity (personal time tracker)
Fantastical (calendar, easy to use, simple phrases turn into calendar events)

Fanurio (time tracking for free lancers)
Freckle (time tracking)
Free-Time (searches, easy to use, simple phrases turn into calendar events)
Google Calendar (color options)
Mailbox (manages emails)
My Minutes (time and task tracker)
Pocket Informant (calendar)
QuickCal Mobile (fast calendar entries)
Re.minder (reminder with notes ability)
Repeat Timer Pro (repeating interval alarm clock timer)
Rescue Time (understand habits to become more focused and productive)
Sunrise (calendar for LinkedIn, pulls profiles into calendar for meetings)
TeuxDeux (task manager with week at a glance view)
TIME Planner (time tracker and productivity enhancer)
Time Sheet (time and work tracking, including expenses and breaks)
Timely (scheduling and time tracking)
Toggl (time tracking)

Word Processing, Drawing, Writing

Byword (text editor with file sharing)
DayOne (for journaling)
Dragon Dictation (dictate: speaking is often quicker than typing)
Google Docs (create and share documents online)
INKredible (note-taking)
NotesPlus (from handwritten notes and images to organized files)
Paper (not word processing but "drawing processing")
Pop (prototyping an app from a piece of paper)
Quip (integrates docs, chat and spreadsheets)

Appendix F: Reducing, Sorting, and Organizing Papers

The guidance that follows helps you whittle down the papers you have and then sort and organize them so that you can get to them when you need to. Contrary to my advice in Chapter 2 to stop in the middle of an action, it is best to start and work through each step only when you have the time to complete that step. Don't try to get through all the steps in one sitting.

The guidance here is explicit and detailed so that you can spend your time on the task at hand and not have to worry about the process.

Step 1: The Initial Sort

Assumptions:

- *Paper is everywhere.*
- *There are different types of papers and documents.*
- *There is no space clear enough to organize them.*

Actions:

- You are clearing off your desk or table for a fresh start.
- Get a big box or basket.
- Dump enough of the paper into the container so that you have a clear space to work.
- Don't look at the papers while you do this, it will slow you down.
- Put the container to one side of the room.
- Get a large trash bag, shake it out so it's ready, and put it to one side of you.
- Take the container and put it on the other side of you.
- Take four index cards and make tents by folding them in half. Label the tents based on the list below and place a tent in each of the "quadrants of the table."

    1. *Important Papers to Store*
    2. *Papers Needing Immediate Action*
    3. *Papers Needing Future Action*
    4. *Papers to File*
    5. *Trash*

The fifth "quadrant" is the trash bag. Anything that is not vital goes there. At this point you can't keep any "maybe papers" or "one day I'll..." papers. You simply are too far behind and have too much paper clutter to have that luxury.

If you don't know what important papers to store, take a look at those listed under File Categories in this appendix and use this as a reference point.

- Begin to sort the papers from the container. Work quickly and efficiently.
- Once you identify what the paper is, put it in the proper pile.
- Don't take the time to fully inspect each paper and get involved with it.
- This is a "down and dirty" sort. Speed is key because you want to move as much paper as possible into the trash. You want to get the papers into manageable piles.
- Do this in one sitting. Remember, fast!

Good job! Now take a break.

Step 2: The Second Sort

Assumptions:

- *There are now 4 piles and the 5th (the trash).*
- *You have a space from which to work that only has the 4 piles.*

Actions:

Take the *Important Papers to Store* and review them to make sure they can't be weeded down any more. If they can, do it now.

Place these important documents in a safe place, whether that is a safe, a bank deposit box, a fireproof box, or in a secret compartment in your teddy bear. It doesn't matter just as long as you are consistent where you store them.

Step 3: Sorting Papers Needing Immediate Action

Do an A, B, C sort of *Papers Needing Immediate Action.*

Actions:
Take these papers and put them in a pile to your side.
Clear the space in front of you so that you have room for three paper piles.
Pick up the top piece of paper from your pile and look at it.

A) Is it super urgent/important?
C) Not very urgent at all/kind of unimportant?
B) Middling between the two?

You will be making piles in front of you. Set the A's to your left, the C's to the right, and the B's directly in front of you.

As you go through the first couple of papers you may be unsure what is an A, B, or C, but as you get going it will become clearer. Now that you have a better handle on how to categorize them, you may need to re-sort the initial few papers, now at the bottom of each pile.

Once you are done with this, go to the A pile and sort those papers in order of importance. If need be, do an a, b, c sort of the A pile (which would become Aa, Ab, Ac). Then stack your papers so that your Aa's—your most important and urgent paper—are on top, your Ab's are next, and your Ac's are on the bottom (that is, descending from the most important and urgent to the still important and urgent, but less so, on the bottom).

During this sort you may have discovered that some of the A's are actually B's. If so remove them from the A pile and put them in the B pile.

Now, sort the B pile in order of importance and urgency. If need be, do a Ba, Bb, and Bc sort.

During this sort you may have discovered that some of the B's are actually C's. If so remove them from the B pile and put them in the C pile.

Pile the B's like you piled the A's, with Ba on top, Bc on the bottom, and Bb in the middle.

Repeat this process with the C pile. Then pile them all together, A's on top, B's in the middle, and C's on the bottom. Put the *Papers Needing Immediate Action* pile aside with the sticky or index card labeling the pile on top.

Step 4: Sorting Papers Needing Future Action

Repeat Step 3, applying this process to the *Papers Needing Future Action* pile, sorting into A, B, C piles (for the C's you don't need to sort them in the Ca, Cb, Cc).

Look at the remaining pile, the C's. Really look at them and then look at the A's and B's, notice how many of them there are, and think about how long it will take you to get through all the A's and B's. Look at the C's again and throw them out. Trash them. You don't have time for them and they aren't important enough to do. By the time you get to them they will be so old that they will be obsolete.

If you must, check quickly for anything dire, but trust me, if they are in the C pile they have outlived their purpose.

You should now have a stacked pile of *Papers Needing Future Action* with the A's on top and B's on the bottom. Put a sticky or index card to label the stacks. This pile goes under the *Papers Needing Immediate Action* pile. Now you have the order for which you start taking action on these papers. Attacking the papers 15 to 30 minutes a day until you get to the bottom of the pile.

The important papers are stored, papers that need immediate and future action in descending order of importance, meaning that you start at the top and work your way down until finished and ready for you to take action. You may now throw out your trash bag of papers.

Now, do a happy dance! But not for long...What is left is the papers to file.

Step 5: Setting Up Categories for Your Files

A classic mistake people affected by ADHD make is creating filing systems so complicated that they never use them. Keep this in mind as you set up your filing system and be sure to keep it simple. Otherwise it's likely you won't use it because you can't remember how you set it up or it just takes too long to file anything.

With that in mind, keep the number of files to a minimum and use the same filing system in your computer files so the filing systems mirror each other.

If possible, keep to one folder per category. Use a subcategory only if the one file folder is too unwieldy. The more you break your files down into subcategories the harder it is to remember where to file items. The fewer files, the more likely you will re-file the item.

For certain documents, keep copies for your files rather than the originals. Keep the originals in a safe deposit box in a bank you have easy access to or in your home in a fireproof box. (You may think that is going to extremes but there was a fire in my home last year.)

Below are some suggested file categories. Use what fits your needs. If you need to create additional files, make sure to keep the categories broad.

File Categories

Bank Records – bank accounts, loans, mortgage or lease records, bank deposit box information, and other banking-related items.

Cars and Other Vehicles – purchase documents, maintenance and service records, insurance, copies of titles.

Children (one set for each child) – school information, important schedules/dates/contacts, educational records, copy of birth certificate, health records, including immunizations

Contacts – names, numbers, address, directions, birthdays, anniversaries, etc. (Don't worry about making this pretty. You won't refer to this file often, so just have a folder and put the information in it. Transfer the information you need to act on to your calendar.)

Financial Records – credit card agreements and perks, investments, paid bills, (File bills as you pay them; they will end up in chronological order, making it easy to search for a bill. Do not make a file for each type of bill. It will deter you from filing the bills.)

Home – copy of title to home, land loan papers, inventory of household items of high value (best to take pictures of these as well), homeowner's or renter's insurance, home repairs and improvements, diagrams or floor plans, warrantees, service plans, and manuals.

Important Papers – (Consider keeping these in a bank safe deposit box.) copy of driver's license, passport (current and expired), wills, birth certificates, divorce papers, military records, adoption papers, titles to vehicles, title to home, death certificates.

Medical and Health Insurance Records – (one file per adult) insurance for health, dental and disability, medical notes, eye prescriptions, immunization records, medication prescriptions. (I recommend keeping a list of your medications and dosages with you at all times in case of emergency; this also helps you fill out forms at the doctor's office easily. It can be an index card in your wallet for example.)

Memberships – any membership whether contracted or not, such as civic organization, health clubs, country clubs, church, professional organizations.

Pets – any related papers such as medical, pet insurance, registration, care instructions for pet sitters.

Taxes – anything related to your taxes such as possible deductions, previous tax returns.

Work Records (one set for each adult) – Social Security information, benefit package, retirement/pension, employment contracts, pay stubs or wage statements, resumes and earned certificates, degrees, and trainings.

Vacations and Travel – Research, plans, and information on vacations and travel, mileage and other rewards information.

How Long to Keep Financial Records

3 Years – records related to filing your income tax, e.g. mortgage statements, charitable contributions, proof of deductible purchases, all business- and income-related documents

7 Years – state and federal income tax returns, real estate tax forms and records, receipts used for tax deductions

Forever – birth certificates, marriage/divorce papers, wills, current insurance policies, education records, pension and retirement plan records, contracts and property agreements

This is the advice I have received from my accountant. Check with your financial advisor or accountant, as your circumstances may require special attention.

About Abigail Wurf, M.Ed, PCC

Abigail Wurf, M.Ed, PCC, founder and president of Abigail Wurf Coaching LLC, specializes in one-on-one and small group coaching. She leads mastermind groups and conducts self-directed programs, webinars, teleseminars, workshops, and speaking engagements. She has given sessions at the national meetings of major organizations in the ADHD field, contributed to three well-received books in the field, serves on the national board of the ADHD Coaches Organization, and now has published *Forget Perfect*.

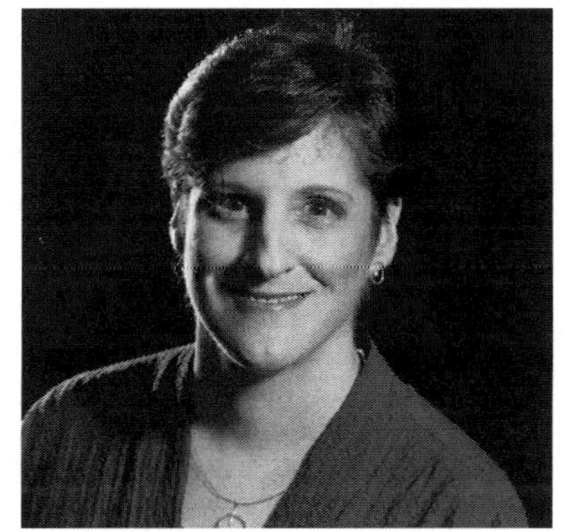

For more than three years she has led monthly meetings at her neighborhood public library for people affected by ADHD. Abigail attributes much of her knowledge to her interaction with the diverse group of people who attend. Her clients credit her with asking strategic questions that motivate them to take action and for having a wonderful sense of humor that helps them deal with tough situations.

Abigail found her first calling in the arts, starting with pre-ballet classes at the age of four. After completing her BA in History, she pursued her passion for the arts as a dancer, choreographer, teacher and co-founder of Arts in Motion in St. Louis, and assistant director of the Mid-America Dance Company. A serious back injury and unsuccessful surgery ended her dance career.

Before returning to study for an advanced degree, she sought an evaluation for learning difficulties and found out that she had ADHD severe enough to fall under the Americans with Disability Act. She earned her M.Ed, learned to manage chronic pain, and sought a second career in the field of coaching, with an emphasis on ADHD.

Abigail Wurf received her Professional Coaching Certificate (PCC) from the International Coaches Federation. She received her Master's in Education at Temple University.

Six years ago, Abigail returned to her home town of Washington, DC and now happily lives within a block of where she grew up.

Acknowledgments

As it takes a community to support a person affected by ADHD, it also takes a community to write a book, especially if the author has ADHD.

This book, much less anything else in my life, would not have been possible if not for two dedicated and talented doctors. Dr. Robert Gerwin upon my first appointment was honest enough to say he didn't know if he could help me with my physical pain. He gave me my life back. The late Dr. Kate Plaisier helped move me from the mental pain of depression, anxiety, and unsuccessfully treated ADHD to what is now a great life. Without these two I would still be dwelling in darkness.

This book is also possible because of the participants in the ADHD Support Group I run and my clients. They have all taught, and will continue to teach, me. We have grown together. A special shout out goes to B. L., one of my first clients, for insisting that I write a book and showing me how to get started on it.

My first coaching mentors, Lynn Meinke and Tina Elliot, helped me understand what coaching was really about. They both pushed me to go deeper and hear what the client really means, not just what the client is saying.

Jodi Sleeper-Triplett trained me in ADHD coaching. I am thankful that I was in the right place at the right time to hear her speak, learn that ADHD coaching existed, and then train with her.

Much thanks goes to Cathi Harley and the rest of the SEC team, including Suzanne Evans herself. They've coached me on keeping Abigail Wurf Coaching, LLC growing so I can reach more people. I can't thank you all enough.

I thank the ADHD coaching community, a group of people dedicated to supporting those affected by ADHD. I must mention in particular Laurie Dupar for the advice and welcome she offered me when I was a newbie and the ADHD Coaches Organization (ACO) Board members, who were there when I joined the board two years ago, especially Sarah Wright, Katherine Jahnke, Joyce Kubik, Terri Gantt, and Virginia Hurley.

I owe a great deal to Anthony Washington for his expertise on just about everything. Thanks for the great photos, my first website, discussions, suggestions, and simply being one of the nicest people I have ever met.

David Cockrell calls me every Tuesday morning to keep me on track and gives great guidance. I thank him for sticking with me.

So many others have helped through training, starting a new business, and finding opportunities. Marcee Rollandini and I met while training to be coaches. We have supported each other as we move forward in our careers and in the unending quest to become better at what we do and who we are. Karen Mulhauser and her tribe of Consulting Women have been a valuable resource for me from the beginning.

I feel it is especially important to acknowledge the doctors and researchers without whose work we wouldn't know that ADHD is both real and manageable: Dr. Edward Hallowell, Dr. John Ratey, Dr. Russell Barkley, and Dr. Thomas Brown, in particular. Their work has not only advanced knowledge of ADHD in medicine and academia, but also increased public awareness of ADHD.

This book would not exist without the hard work of my editor, Cathy Kreyche. I am glad our worlds collided. I don't think there could be a better fit for me to help me through this process.

I did well in the brother department. My brother Nick asks questions that cut to the heart of the matter, and he is there to offer advice and support whenever I ask for it. My mother, to whom this book is dedicated, has put in countless hours towards getting this book done. Whether editing my writing, answering my questions, or just being patient with me while keeping me on task, she has gone well beyond the call of duty. To use her words, I am glad she is a part of my "posse."

Made in the USA
Middletown, DE
06 June 2015